Experientia
Treatm
for PTS

The Therapeutic Spiral Model

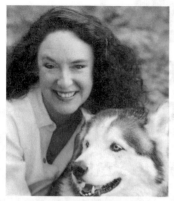

Kate Hudgins, PhD, is a clinical psychologist and board certified trainer in psychodrama, sociometry and group psychotherapy. She received the 2001 Innovator's Award from the American Society of Group Psychotherapy and Psychodrama for creating The Therapeutic Spiral Model, which integrates classical psychodrama with recent clinical advances in trauma practice and training. She established the nonprofit organization Therapeutic Spiral International in 2000 to bring this model of healing to underserved areas of the global community. She is a published author whose work includes *Psychodrama with Trauma Survivors: Acting Out Your Pain* (2002). Kate travels extensively and has trained Action Trauma Teams in Australia, Canada, England, New Zealand, Northern Ireland, and South Africa, and has taught in many additional countries including Israel, South Korea, and Turkey.

Experiential Treatment for PTSD

The Therapeutic Spiral Model

M. Katherine Hudgins, PhD, TEP

 Springer Publishing Company

Springer Publishing Company, Inc.
536 Broadway
New York, NY 10012-3955

Acquisitions Editor: Sheri W. Sussman
Production Editor: Jeanne W. Libby
Cover design by Joanne E. Honigman

01 02 03 04 05/5 4 3 2 1

Library of Congress Cataloging-in-Publication Data

Hudgins, Kate, 1953–
   Experiential treatment for PTSD : the therapeutic spiral model / M. Katherine Hudgins.
      p. ; cm.
   Includes bibliographical references and index.
   ISBN 0-8261-4942-1
   1. Psychodrama.   2. Post-traumatic stress disorder—Treatment.   I. Title.
   [DNLM: 1. Psychodrama—methods.   2. Stress Disorders,
   Post-Traumatic—therapy.
WM 430.5.P8 H884t 2002]
RC489.P7.H833 2002
616.85'21—dc21
                                                            2002017742
                                                            CIP

Printed in the United States of America by Capital City Press.

Contents

Preface

> Experiencing trauma is an essential part of being human:
> History is written in blood. (van der Kolk and McFarlane,
> 1996, p. 3)

Trauma is inescapable in today's world. It is heard in the violent sounds of guns that rage, student to student, in U.S. high schools. It's seen in the sad and frightened eyes of a battered woman. It permeates the news media that surround us all.

On September 11th, 2001, we all experienced trauma in ways we could not believe were possible until that moment. This book, and the method of treating posttraumatic stress disorder (PTSD) that it teaches, the Therapeutic Spiral Model, was created before "9/11." As PTSD reaches epidemic numbers among peoples around the world, it is my hope that the words here can make a difference.

For the purposes of this handbook, trauma is defined as the result of any single experience or ongoing experience that felt life-threatening and broke through normal coping mechanisms. Overpowering events overwhelm the ability to defend against pain, loss, and possible death. Cognitive processes are frozen in time as the self tries to cope with intense emotions in the face of a real danger that made no sense. In everyday language, trauma is the feeling that everything is spiraling out of control and there is no way to make it stop.

POSTTRAUMATIC STRESS DISORDER

In the early 1980s several changes in the way mental health problems were viewed became evident. The American Psychiatric Association (APA) recognized that the "war neuroses" of Vietnam veterans were, in fact, a stress-induced disorder. Today, the *DSM-IV-TR* (*Diagnostic and Statistical Manual of Mental Disorders-Revised*, 2000) defines PTSD as a problem experienced by 1 out of 10 people from a variety of stressors (see Appendix A).

Since that time, PTSD has become an internationally recognized problem, in the face of earthquakes; school shootings; random violence; addiction; ethnic tension; and war and torture of individuals, groups, and cultures. Psychologists, therapists, refugee and aid workers, advocates, and relief organizations seek fast and effective intervention at the time of natural and social catastrophe.

It is expected that 70% of the people who experienced and/or witnessed the recent terrorist attacks on the USA will show signs of posttraumatic stress. Of these, 20% will go on to develop the disorder of PTSD 6 months after the events. With the expected increase of PTSD in the wake of these acts of terror, we need quicker and more effective treatments that address the core of trauma experiences, not just the symptoms they cause.

Over the past 10 years, active methods of change have come to the fore to treat all stress-induced disorders. Grassroots groups, such as self-help, 12-step groups embrace experiential methods in inpatient treatment for addictions and eating disorders. Advances in psychotherapy research show experiential methods can treat trauma effectively and more efficiently than talk therapy.

EXPERIENTIAL TREATMENT OF PTSD

My first exposure to the treatment of PTSD using experiential methods was during my NIMH (National Institute for Mental Health) internship in psychodrama and group psychotherapy at St. Elizabeth's Hospital, in Washington, D.C., in the early 1980s. I was practicing my skills as a new psychodrama director with my peer group of other interns. We had been having a group conflict, so I told the group to "take their imaginary guns, build their camps, and set up the battle lines"—enacting a group metaphor to make the covert overt. All went well with the loud noises of guns, much shouting, and even a few jokes. It seemed the action structure was helping people to express anger in a safe and playful manner.

All of a sudden, one of my peers, a Vietnam veteran, started to experience body memories. He was flooded by intense dissociated feelings. He fell to his knees. He was unconsciously reexperiencing a flashback to the war. I was stunned. I had never witnessed a flashback in the calm confines of talk therapy. We were all, in his experience of the moment, unequivocably *in* Vietnam. Our stage had become the jungle, and there were dead bodies of women and children around him. I looked at my supervisor and said, "What do I do now?" She replied, "Direct the drama."

Taking a deep breath, I did direct the drama. As a healing community we walked the jungles with the veteran, gathering up and burying the wounds of his past—the men, women, and children he put in a psychodramatic grave. The minister in our group did a blessing and burial. We joined him in his keel of grief. Time shifted again.

As fellow students, we returned to the here and now of the training group and looked around the psychodrama stage. We held hands, wept and sang with him, integrating him back into our community. Now we, too, directly shared his knowledge of the experience of the horror and pain of war, and, most importantly, we all experienced healing.

I was touched with the power of classical psychodrama to truly heal deep psychological wounds that day. I was also scared as a new therapist to use these same methods, for fear of triggering uncontrolled regression and out-of-control affect. Somehow that day, the seeds of a clinically modified model of psychodrama with trauma began to take root in my mind. After completing my PhD in clinical psychology, becoming a Board Certified Psychodrama Trainer, and practicing as a therapist and trainer with trauma survivors for over 20 years, the harvest is in.

This book introduces both practitioners and trainers to the Therapeutic Spiral Model (TSM). TSM is a clinical system of experiential change to heal trauma induced by any overpowering life circumstance. It integrates theoretical foundations from neurobiology, self-psychology, object relations theory, experiential therapy research, and the methods of classical psychodrama. Client stories are shared and put into action to demonstrate the heart and art of the Therapeutic Spiral Model.

My hope by sharing this action method in writing is to reach a greater number of people who work with and/or have experienced trauma themselves. It could not be more timely.

VOICES OF SURVIVORS

Although many people have given permission to share their personal recovery with the Therapeutic Spiral Model, our "clients" do not use their real names. I have created composites of the people whom I have been privileged to work with in my years of clinical practice. Their stories demonstrate what is normal for many trauma survivors when trauma strikes—and when life is restored to a place of trust in self and others. Let me introduce the clients who will share their stories throughout this handbook.

Tricia brings a story of healing from childhood sexual abuse. The abuse happened in a wealthy American family who seemed to "have it all." On the outside she looked good—successful, powerful, and intelligent. Inside, she was consumed by body memories, intrusive feelings, and uncontrolled reexperiencing of childhood sexual abuse. She was referred to me because her work as a defense attorney was suffering. We worked together for nearly a year in individual therapy, and she attended quarterly weekend workshops using the Therapeutic Spiral Model. Today, Tricia is in complete remission from her chronic symptoms of PTSD, even when stressed by her career.

Vladimir is a 27-year-old Serbian psychologist who was a counselor at a refugee center in Australia. He immigrated to Sydney in 1994, fleeing the civil war in former Yugoslavia. He left behind his entire childhood family, not knowing whether they were dead or alive. He learned TSM in a 2-year training program on using action methods with refugees. Vladamir states that TSM provided him with the strength to begin again in a new place after his many losses, and most of all to restore hope for his future. He then carried what he had learned about TSM with trauma survivors to his refugee clients.

Jim is a 50-year-old recovering alcoholic, who works as the head counselor at a halfway house in upstate New York. When he began to attend TSM workshops as an adjunct to his recovery process, he had been sober for 9 years. However, he was still haunted by his childhood in an abusive, violent, alcoholic home. He often reexperienced body memories of being hit with canes, belts, and once burned with scalding water. He had nightmares and flashbacks several times a week. He was divorced, lonely, and without hope. After integrating six intensive weekends with his individual therapy, he was able to make peace with his past.

Andrea came into TSM therapy a 20-year-old anorexic woman who was gang-raped in college and had gone into a suicidal depression in her freshman year. She participated in intensive individual and group treatment for 8 months using TSM. She attended quarterly workshops for 2 years and made a full recovery from her eating disorder. At 30, she now has a productive life that includes work as an architect, a good marriage, and a lively 3-year-old daughter.

A PERSONAL NOTE

This book has taken many years to write. A lot has happened in the decade during which I developed and practiced this model with action trauma teams around the world. To help support team building in under-resourced communities, I opened Therapeutic Spiral International (TSI), a nonprofit organization, in 2000. Our mission is to provide experiential education, training, and direct services to people effected by trauma in the global community. TSI is the sponsor of the Postgraduate Accreditation Program in the Therapeutic Spiral Model.

My original purpose in writing this book was to convey to health professionals the depth of change possible for traumatized people using experiential methods of change. Today, 6 months after the beginning of terrorist attacks in America, my purpose is also to bring hope to the hearts of practitioners who work with trauma survivors at this time of greatest need. Now is the time that PTSD can be diagnosed after the acts of terror on September 11th, 2001. Now is the time that treatment can make a difference in people's lives. Take what you can from this book and use it for yourself and your clients.

As you read this book, I ask you to pace yourself. Four clients share their unspeakable horrors with you in word and action. If you feel emotionally overwhelmed and like you are zoning out, take a break and notice what you are responding to in the book. Integrate your learning as you read.

Acknowledgments

I want to personally thank the many protagonists who have shared their stories of trauma and healing with me. Our action trauma teams have worked with people in Australia, Canada, Cyprus, England, South Korea, Northern Ireland, Israel, New Zealand, South Africa, the former Yugoslavia, Turkey, and the U.S.A. in 15 years of TSM training and practice. Thank you for sharing the unspeakable horrors you experienced in the face of family violence and global conflicts. Together, we found ways to understand, express, and heal from the traumas of being human.

I also thank the team members for your dedication and courage. Eyes wide open, you have been witness to stories of horror beyond belief. You have given freely of your hearts and souls. Together, we have created many sacred spaces for deep healing to occur. It has been wonderful to share the journey with other professionals.

I have been blessed to have experienced the support of several extraordinary mentors in my work. Thanks to Zerka T. Moreno for your love and belief in me. Thanks to Dr. Dale Richard Buchanan, psychodrama trainer par excellence! And to Dr. Donald J. Kiesler who guided me through my Ph.D. at Virginia Commonwealth University.

Deep appreciation goes to my husband Peter Dummett for his unwavering love and support. Thanks to Robert Alexander for teaching me about the process of writing and the patience involved. My gratitude to Mimi Cox, Gerry Hanlon, Helen Estoque Hopper, Kathy Metcalf, and others who loved me through it all. Thanks to my son Wes McLaughlin who keeps challenging my mind with his own. And I must not forget my animal companion of 10 years, Mr. Magic, a blue-eyed Siberian husky—thank you for your constant companionship by my side, in my heart, and under my desk.

The Therapeutic Spiral Model™:
An Action Solution to Treating PTSD

The Therapeutic Spiral Model (TSM) was developed to provide a clinical map for therapists working on issues of severe traumatization with clients, regardless of the etiology of the stressor. The TSM defines clear clinical action structures and advanced intervention modules for using experiential methods safely with trauma survivors. In this way, the pace and intensity of classical psychodrama is modified and can be clinically guided, so that regression is controlled, conscious, and always in the service of the ego.

The Therapeutic Spiral Model was developed over 20 years of clinical and training practice using experiential methods with survivors of severe sexual and physical abuse. Since 1995, it has been used with political refugees who in many cases experienced war, imprisonment, torture, and other acts of terror. One of our teams responded to the need for grief counseling for the practitioners in New York City who were supporting the employees of the World Trade Center and their families. In many cases, these clients came to therapy, physically exhausted, emotionally confused, and spiritually bereft.

EXPERIENTIAL PSYCHOTHERAPY

At first glance, the use of psychodramatic methods with trauma survivors may appear rather surprising to many readers. Some of you may have seen the explosive emotions and ego state shifts that can occur in the hands of untrained practitioners using action methods. On the other hand, many of you have personal testimony of healing with experiential methods from family and friends. In fact, there is much to suggest that experiential therapy is a treatment of choice for clients working on a history of trauma when guided from a clinical framework such as the Therapeutic Spiral Model.

Cognitive behavioral therapy has long proved useful in managing the disruptive symptoms of PTSD, but it does not directly treat the core trauma that causes these very symptoms. In fact, in many veteran hospitals and addiction centers, counselors shy away from addressing the core trauma, only to find that their clients continue to have flashbacks and nightmares that trigger relapses. Conversely, experiential therapies directly target the disrupted and disorganized self-structures for true developmental repair.

CLASSICAL PSYCHODRAMA

Developed in the early 1900s by physician J. L. Moreno and his wife and partner Zerka, classical psychodrama is the seminal method of experiential therapy (Blatner, 2000; Fox, 1987). Psychodrama started out as a form of therapeutic theater and over the past 75 years has evolved more and more into a clinically effective method of therapy and behavior change. Most importantly, psychodrama structures the telling of one's story in ways that people with PTSD find useful and healing.

> There is in psychodrama a mode of experience, which goes beyond reality, which provides the subject with a new and more extensive experience of reality, a surplus reality. (Moreno, J. L., 1965, p. 212)

Surplus Reality

It is, in fact, this "surplus reality" that trauma survivors live in on a daily basis. Flashbacks from the past interrupt the present moment. Body memories crash through during moments of intimacy. Feelings of being a little child in an adult's body are frequent. People with PTSD often have a sense of simultaneously inhabiting two worlds—the "real," outside world and what is occurring in it, and a world comprised of the happenings inside them: their thoughts, feelings, and reactions.

Classical psychodrama allows people to share the chaos of their internal world in a group setting. Methods of surplus reality bring both inner and outer worlds of experience together at the same time

(Holmes, 1992; Moreno, Blomqvist, & Rützel, 2000). It is a powerful method of therapeutic change for all people.

As seen with my first directing experience of a Vietnam veteran, however, classical psychodrama also has the potential for uncontrolled regression, and unfortunately, even retraumatization when working with vulnerable clients. Sometimes these difficulties result from poorly trained therapists who take one or two experiential workshops and use these powerful methods inappropriately or worse. Even seasoned psychodramatists, Gestalt therapists, and others question how to use action methods safely with trauma survivors. The Therapeutic Spiral Model was created from a clinician's perspective to guide classical psychodrama and to provide answers to questions that might arise.

THE THERAPEUTIC SPIRAL MODEL TO TREAT TRAUMA

As an experiential method, the Therapeutic Spiral Model increases treatment effectiveness while decreasing treatment time with PTSD. Practitioners discover techniques to provide containment and safety with action methods in educational, community, and therapeutic settings. Clients find a method that understands the chaos of their internal world and helps them find ways to express it.

The Therapeutic Spiral Model intends to provide the following:

1. client-friendly constructs that explain internal, self-organization for trauma survivors;
2. clear clinical action structures for safe experiential practice with trauma survivors; and
3. advanced action intervention modules for containment, expression, repair, and integration of unprocessed trauma material.

STRUCTURE OF THE BOOK

This book follows a written structure that includes theory, practice, and clinical processing. Each chapter contains action vignettes and case examples to demonstrate the methods of the Therapeutic Spiral Model. Clients guide us in understanding and experiencing the power of experiential methods, when clinically directed.

Part I (chapters 1–3) presents the theoretical foundations of the Therapeutic Spiral Model.

Chapter 1 presents the latest research and theories on the physical nature of trauma. Neurobiology details brain research showing that trauma is stored in the nonverbal, emotional centers of the brain—which are not accessible in talk therapy. Self-psychology and object relations theory describe how trauma impacts psychological self-organization and social, interpersonal relationships.

Chapter 2 presents the theory and research of experiential psychotherapy. Recently shown to be as effective as cognitive behavioral and psychodynamic therapy, it is becoming a treatment of choice for trauma survivors. Classical psychodrama is the foundation of the Therapeutic Spiral Model. A discussion on the pitfalls of action methods is also included.

Chapter 3 introduces the Therapeutic Spiral Model to treat PTSD using experiential methods. Energy, experiencing, and meaning make up the three strands of the spiral. The therapeutic spiral is the first TSM clinical action structure to guide clinical decision making with trauma survivors.

Part II (chapters 4–6) presents three additional clinical action structures of the Therapeutic Spiral Model and provides the experiences shared by our clinical guides.

Chapter 4 describes the use of a trained action trauma team. The roles of team leader, assistant leader, and trained auxiliary egos are defined and demonstrated. Their functions as analyst, therapist, sociometrist, and producer are presented and discussed.

Chapter 5 details the trauma survivor's intrapsychic role atom. This clinical map uses role theory to guide all action interventions in the Therapeutic Spiral Model. Prescriptive, trauma-based, and transformative roles make up the role atom that guides clinical implementation of experiential interventions.

Chapter 6 presents the types of reexperiencing dramas in the Therapeutic Spiral Model. There are six types of dramas, each with their own clinical contract and action structures.

Part III (chapters 7–10) demonstrates the Therapeutic Spiral Model in action and practice. The final two clinical action structures are presented through a clinical example in chapters 7 and 8. Clinical processing of the session is completed in chapters 9 and 10.

Chapter 7 describes the first two scenes in a TSM drama for conscious reexperiencing and developmental repair. The prescriptive roles and the defensive structures are demonstrated. Interventions of restoration, observation, and containment teach clients to hold traumatic experience in present awareness and without primitive defenses, such as denial, dissociation, and projective identification.

Chapter 8 completes the TSM drama of conscious reexperiencing and developmental repair. Scenes 3, 4, and 5 show the safe enactment of trauma-based roles; in this example, the victim role. Scene 6 shows the power of developmental repair using the Therapeutic Spiral Model.

Chapter 9 begins the clinical processing of the TSM drama detailed in the previous two chapters. Scenes 1 and 2 are discussed, with a director's soliloquy. Intervention modules for restorative roles, the observing ego, the body double, the containing double, and the manager of healthy functioning are all detailed.

Chapter 10 completes the clinical processing of the TSM drama for conscious reexperiencing and developmental repair. Intervention modules for the safe enactment of trauma-based roles and the client role are detailed. The step-by-step process for controlled regression and conscious abreaction is demonstrated.

Part IV (chapters 10–12) completes the book with a look at training, research, and future projections.

Chapter 11 presents the TSM team process to prevent secondary posttraumatic stress disorder in practitioners working with trauma. Team support and a commitment to rigorous honesty among team members builds a container for debriefing and one's own letting go.

Chapter 12 shares the recent application of the Therapeutic Spiral Model outside the therapeutic setting. Joining together with humanities scholars, the TSM has been adapted for public education and community programs about PTSD, following the attacks on 911. It also presents research on TSM and summarizes the effectiveness of the work across settings.

Enjoy the reading. At this time of uncertainty and fear in the world, I hope it feeds your mind with ideas, theories, and methods of practice. I hope it touches your heart, through the warmth and beauty of scenes of trust and healing. I hope it helps you to reach out to others, to help us all have new and fortifying experiences in today's world, so that trauma is no longer a defining human experience.

Kate

April 2002

PART ONE

Trauma and Experiential Therapy

The first section of this book presents the theoretical foundations of the Therapeutic Spiral Model. While the clinical action structures and the advanced intervention modules give practitioners new tools to work with clients, it is the integrated clinical theory that provides the basis for safety in TSM.

Chapter 1 details the present understanding of the effects of overwhelming stress on people. Many advances have been made over the past decade in the fields of neurobiology, self-psychology, and object relations theory. The Therapeutic Spiral Model organizes these theories so they guide the clinical practice of experiential methods of change.

Chapter 2 prescribes experiential therapy as a treatment of choice for PTSD with its nonverbal symptoms. The principles of change that guide TSM are active experiencing, adaptive use of affect, and regression in the service of the ego. Classical psychodrama is modified by the clinical theories above to provide safe experiential treatment for trauma in the Therapeutic Spiral Model.

The final chapter in this section presents the first clinical action structure, the spiral image, that guides clinical practice in the Therapeutic Spiral Model, drawing together the theories of the first two chapters.

CHAPTER ONE

The Experiential Impact of Trauma

CHAPTER OVERVIEW

Traumatic events, such as those of 911, impact deeply and profoundly how peoples and cultures experience themselves and the world around them. Personal assumptions of safety and connection are shaken at their roots. The rules for being in the world change whenever trauma happens. Trauma is basic and life changing to all who experience it.

As stated in the *Preface*, this book uses the DSM-IV-TR diagnosis of posttraumatic stress disorder to begin to understand the complex symptoms shown by many survivors of trauma. This medical diagnosis does not even come close, however, to describing the full experience of trauma on body, mind, emotions, and spirit.

To help the reader understand the pervasive impact of trauma better, this chapter also discusses several theories, that will provide a foundation of knowledge about trauma:

- neurobiology,
- self psychology, and
- object relations theory.

Then these theories are integrated into a client-friendly concept—a graphic description of the experience of trauma. "Trauma bubbles" help bridge the gap between the nonverbal symptoms of PTSD and the words to describe them.

Even psychologically sophisticated clients have a hard time communicating the often unseen distress of posttraumatic stress. They experience unpredictable cycles of numbness and intensity. They report "feeling like I'm going crazy," "not being in my body," and "feeling like a 3-year-old child." Many clients find themselves caught in the throws of addictions and eating disorders in vain attempts to control the disruptive aftermath of trauma.

Listen to Vladamir describe, a year later, how his whole world changed when he had to flee former Yugoslavia due to civil war and ethnic violence:

> I was a successful psychologist at home. I felt I contributed to others. I helped them deal with depression, family problems, and political strife. Now, I am the one who is depressed. I came to Australia to start a new life, but my new life hasn't begun yet.
>
> I am living in the past and I am helpless to change it. When I lie in bed at night, I hear the voice of my mother screaming for me to help her . . . to stop the soldiers from dragging her off. I am sure they raped her and my sisters . . . and then killed them . . . I cannot bear the pain.

DEFINITION OF TRAUMA

Terr's (1991) definition of trauma is the one I have found most useful in my work with survivors of trauma: Trauma is "an (external) blow or series of blows rendering the person temporarily helpless and breaking past ordinary coping and defensive operations" (p. 12).

I chose this definition because it describes trauma regardless of etiology; and thus avoids many of the controversial political and social issues that surround the definition of trauma in the global community. This definition applies to both children and adults. It is inclusive and based on how the person actually experienced a traumatic situation, not on what stressor caused the event.

EXPERIENTIAL DEFINITION OF SELF

For the purposes of this book, a current definition of self that is from an experiential view of personality is employed. As Greenberg and Van Balen (1998) state,

> The term "self" refers not to an entity but to the tacit level of organization that acts as the integrating agent of experience that separates what is me from what is not me. (p. 44)

As a clinical psychologist, I found this flexible, in-the-moment definition of self to be the most helpful in working with trauma survivors. It relates directly to one's level of functioning in the here and now. It frames ego states as normal and responsive to change. Self-organization is ever changing, incorporating new information and finding increased meaning making to guide the future.

TRAUMATIC CHANGES IN SELF-ORGANIZATION

When trauma hits, the self becomes psychologically disorganized. The patterns and structures of self-organization that were there, whether in childhood or as an adult, become frozen in time. Violence threatens the very existence of self physically, intellectually, psychologically, emotionally, and spiritually.

Strong defenses form against such terror and pain. Survival modes of living become locked into trauma bubbles in the face of life-threatening experiences. Unfortunately, these survival modes become automatic and continue to be practiced unconsciously many years after trauma ends. Emotions are numb or explosive. Interpersonal connections are fragile, all to protect the self from further hurt.

For therapists and clients alike, it is important to have words to describe these systemic changes in self-organization that happen with trauma. It is the beginning of the cognitive component of the psychological container that supports experiential work with the TSM.

NEUROBIOLOGICAL CHANGES

In the past 10 years, Bessel van der Kolk, a noted Harvard researcher, and his colleagues have transformed the understanding of the body's map of trauma. While most therapists can tell you that the "body remembers what the mind forgets," neuroscientists are now showing physical, measurable, biochemical changes in the brains of people who have experienced trauma (van der Kolk, 1996a, 1996b, 1997a).

Empirical research studies using MRIs and other advanced brain imaging techniques show that unprocessed trauma experiences are held in neurochemical brain structures related to emotional processing of information (van der Kolk, McFarlane, & Weisaeth, 1996). Thus, research in neurobiology shows that flashbacks and body memories, common PTSD symptoms, activate the emotional but not cognitive parts of the brain. Even dissociation has been shown to have biochemical correlates in the brain (van der Kolk, van der Hart, & Marmar, 1996).

We now know that the frontal cortex, the center of cognitive functioning in humans, is not activated when traumatic memories are reexperienced in experimental settings. Sensory and perceptual lenses are affected at the neurological level. Trauma survivors actually *do* see the world differently.

No wonder trauma survivors say they cannot make sense of their traumatic experiences. Literally, there are no words. Brains impacted by trauma are unable to put meaning to unprocessed experiences. These fragmented memories are then stored in the right brain and organized around affect, not words. Neurobiological research gives credence to the many personal stories of what it feels like to be a trauma survivor.

Perceptual distortions, intense dissociated feelings, body memories, flashbacks, primitive defenses, ego state changes and even unconscious repetitions of early trauma can haunt any survivor of trauma (Ellenson, 1986, 1989; Gelinas, 1983; Young, 1992). Intimate relationships are fraught with difficulties and transference becomes the veil though which the present is experienced (Courtois, 1988). The inner world becomes unsafe—and remains so long after the actual traumatic incident has ended in the outer world.

For years Jim explained the flashbacks and body memories of his violent childhood as the result of his alcoholic drinking. After 9 years of sobriety, however, he was still waking up in the night screaming, sweating, and shaking like a little boy. As Jim described himself to his addictions counselor,

> I used to think I "saw things" because I was so drunk I was hallucinating. But ya know, I've been clean and sober for almost 10 years now . . . and I still see and hear things that aren't "there"—most everyday.
>
> Sometimes, I hear my father's voice screaming at me that I am worthless, no good, not wanted. I can see the rage and hatred in my father's eyes looking out at me when I look in the mirror to shave. It's like time shifts and I know my body is in this room, but it feels like I am hiding in the living room of the house I grew up in. Scares me to death sometimes.

CHANGES IN SELF-PERCEPTION

Rather than feeling vital and effective in the world, many trauma survivors withdraw and rely on avoidance and isolation to stay safe (Bass & Davis, 1988). They lose a sense of resiliency when so much energy is used to manage unprocessed trauma experience and dissociated emotions. Those in intimate relationships have all sorts of difficulties with both attachment and separation (Dayton, 1997; Herman, 1992a, 1992b).

A year after she was gang-raped, Andrea said in a session with me,

> I used to be this lively, happy girl, ready to take on the world. I was so excited about starting college and moving out from Mom and Dad. I was almost valedictorian at my high school and I was poplar with the boys. I knew good things were ahead of me. But now . . .
>
> Now, I am a scared, lonely, and ugly girl inside and out. I go to school still, but I don't care about it anymore. I have no ambition. My grades suck. All I care about is being left alone so I can be safe.
>
> My beautiful silver scales, that is what matters to me now. I can control the number on the scale and that makes me happy. I can get on the scale 100 times a day just to see if I am the same weight. Except for school I rarely leave my apartment.
>
> I hate my life now.

As is obvious, Andrea's whole self-concept changed when she was sexually assaulted. A year later, she suffered from anorexia in a vain attempt to control her feelings. Trauma does, as we see, cause changes in thinking, feeling, defenses, and relationships.

CHANGES IN THINKING

When trauma happens, information processing regresses to the preverbal level because intense emotions overwhelm thinking. Cognitive structures are compromised through physiological pain, psychological vulnerability, and the emotional intensity of terror. "Losing my mind" is an accurate description of what horror feels like during any experience of trauma. When emotions overwhelm thinking, traumatic experience does not simply go away. It becomes stored, without words, in the emotional centers of the right brain.

Sensorimotor Representation

Unprocessed memories of trauma are fragmented and free floating in unconscious awareness. Images are split apart. Sounds and smells hold feelings of terror and horror. Intense grief and rage are dissociated.

The pieces of reality are not labeled. They are not accessible by words. This way of thinking is called sensorimotor representation. It is how the brain works prior to the ability to put words to experience. It is also how the brain experiences trauma. It means that the unconscious trauma material is experienced as sensations, nonverbal behaviors, and emotional tones. There are no words attached to the representations. Clients experience flashes of images, sensations, feelings, urges for action, but they don't know what they all mean.

Jim says that anytime he smells alcohol now, he also sees his father's face raging at him. Andrea shares how she looks over her shoulder at least 50 times a day because she feels someone breathing on her neck, even when she is locked in her apartment alone. Vladamir stands in the line at the supermarket and dives to the floor when he hears what he thinks is the sound of gunfire, as a car backfires in the parking lot. Tricia experiences flashbacks of hands and hostility, while sitting at her desk preparing for court.

Obsessional Patterns

Rigid, compartmentalized, and repetitive patterns of thinking may also develop in an attempt to control unprocessed trauma material. Many people do this through socially acceptable compulsions like work and exercise. Others end up with obsessive compulsive disorders and addictions that fully debilitate their lives (Dayton, 2000).

Tricia was 34 years old when she started therapy. She was a successful attorney who was married to her third husband, a man with inherited wealth and an interest in the arts. She easily worked all day, every day of the week, as a criminal defense advocate at a prestigious law firm in a big U.S. city. Her life was filled with intellectual stimulation, fast-paced meetings, long hours, and high status. She often said she was happy now—after two failed marriages and continued emotional distance from her only child.

Internally, however, Tricia was still tormented by shattered images of herself as a child. Try as she did with her workaholic lifestyle, she could not blot out the nightmares that would wake her, screaming in terror, in the middle of the night. Her husband would hold and soothe her. She would calm down on the outside, but inside she couldn't stop the voices from screaming over and over again, in words she did not understand.

Both sensorimotor representation and the obsessional thinking it generates are a normal part of the aftermath of trauma. Giving words to these symptoms can make a great difference to survivors trying to understand themselves. They are not crazy. It's just how their mind manifests experiences until there are words to describe unprocessed events.

CHANGES IN EMOTION

"In a sense, feelings are ultimately the meeting place of mind, body, environment, culture, and behavior" (Greenberg, Rice, & Elliott, 1993, p. 54). Recent research in emotion theory shows the following: a) the primacy of adaptive affects, b) the rich interplay of cognition and emotions in healthy functioning, and c) the organizing nature of emotions (Greenberg & Pavio, 1997).

All memories are organized around primary affects—emotions that are experienced as a general level of arousal and awareness. In healthy development, the organizing feelings become safety, connection, and self-motivation.

Emotional Intensity

In the case of traumatic memory, the organizing feelings become terror, horror, disgust, helplessness, shame, rage, despair, and/or grief (Greenberg & Pavio, 1998). Experiencing these emotions overwhelms cognitive abilities. Intense affects are then denied, dissociated, or projected out of awareness. These unconscious feelings continue to organize experience in the survivor's life, however, making every event seem fearful and everyone a threat.

The coercive and/or life-threatening nature of many traumas often makes expression of these normal feelings dangerous, both during and after violence. When feelings are too terrible to bear and unable to be expressed, they split off from awareness to protect the core self. Rigid boundaries form between emotional experiencing and expression. Some survivors even develop different personality states to cope with terror, humiliation, and rage. Others give up feeling at all.

Jim's violent father made sure that none of his five kids talked to anyone about the beatings, the thrown and broken objects, and the rages after his drinking. He threatened to kill all of them if any one of them told. So all remained silent not only to protect themselves, but also to save each other.

These intense emotions are experienced in the body when they do get out of their compartments in the mind. They are illustrated by descriptions such as "covered in shame," "sucked under by despair," and "hate so hot it can kill." No wonder people want to push feelings out of awareness, both at the time of trauma and in its wake.

Cycles of Emotions

When traumatic experience happens the body responds to the threat of overwhelming affect by the physiological fight or flight response. PTSD by definition includes alternating cycles of intrusive emotions and fragmented memories with periods of emotional numbness and avoidance of all associations to trauma.

Psychic Numbing.   As mentioned, many trauma survivors turn to substances, eating disorders, and other compulsions to block out the intensity of their unprocessed feelings (Dayton, 2000). Other people numb themselves by avoidance, isolation, and rigid control of their feelings and relationships. No matter how it happens, people with PTSD want the experience of their emotions to become muted, to go away.

Jim talked about how he used alcohol to cope with his flashbacks, only to become an alcoholic. Tricia tried to blot out her past through work and exercise until a case triggered flashbacks. Andrea denied not only her feelings but all body sensations with her anorexia:

> I am like the walking dead. I get up. I go to school. I come home. I have no friends. I don't relate to anyone anymore. I tried to be intimate with a guy I started to like, but every time he even tried to kiss me, I felt like I was about 4 years old. I started crying and shaking. I was so ashamed, so I just don't "have" feelings anymore. It's simpler that way. Just me and my scales.

Emotional Flooding.   These dissociated and denied emotions can be defended against—until some unpredictable cue triggers them in the present. Intense feelings from the past crash through into present relationships, work settings, and time alone. Confusion about past and present can occur in relationships when emotional flooding and ego state changes happen.

Tricia experienced bouts of free-floating rage during the time she was trying the case that first triggered her PTSD symptoms. She stated,

> I would fly into a rage at Bill at home for saying hello some days. No matter how loving he was, I just hated him. I did *not* want him to touch me. I was disgusted, disgusting, and out of control with my anger.
>
> Even at work, I would get out of hand. My poor secretary got a mouthful more than once for honest mistakes. When I was preparing for the opening argument, I must have yelled at every other attorney in our firm on one day or another. I mean, I have always had a temper but this was too much. I didn't even know myself.

Both psychic numbing and emotional flooding impact people's lives on a daily basis as part of PTSD. Being able to understand, and to have words to describe what is happening helps to accurately label emotional experiences for further processing.

CHANGES IN DEFENSIVE STRUCTURES

At the time of trauma, primitive defenses automatically protect the self from experiencing the intense affects of violence. Defenses lock the unprocessed experience into unconscious awareness, waiting for a time when it can be accessed and integrated into cognitive functioning. While protection was needed during the trauma, these same defenses often become automatic long after the event.

Primitive Defenses

Functional amnesia and denial are the mind's way of totally shutting out, forgetting, and not knowing that parts of a traumatic experience happened. Amnesia for entire events can happen as a result of any trauma, but seems to be more prevalent when the violence was chronic and repeated. Andrea is unable to remember much of the gang rape she experienced, and tries to forget what she does recall with her fixation on the numbers on her scale.

Dissociation is the mind's way to split off sensorimotor representations that are too intense to bear. There is a vague sense that there is something disturbing behind the dissociation, but the feelings cannot be accessed through words. Vladamir unconsciously relied on dissociation when triggered in the present. He would sit, stunned, staring out into space, not realizing where he was.

Multiple states of consciousness can form as a defense against extreme violence that is repeated. When this happens, the ego begins to organize states around different feelings. As these states are reinforced by lived experience, they can even develop into personalities if the violence is prolonged.

For many trauma survivors, there are multiple states of consciousness—a child state, a perpetrator state, an adult state, but without the extreme division of personalities. Jim reported the dual states of adult and child on a regular basis, even after 9 years of sobriety.

Idealization is a common interpersonal defense that many trauma survivors use. Because they feel so full of shame themselves, they project their positive feelings onto someone else. They see a person in their lives as all perfect, all knowing, and wonderful, and that reflects back on self. Tricia had idealized her father, a powerful, intelligent, charismatic businessman. In this way she blocked out her feelings about the fact that he also sexually abused her.

Identification with the aggressor is a result of introjecting the representation of the perpetrator and then acting it out toward self or others. Vladamir had unfortunately taken on the defense of identifying with the aggressor as he perpetrated violence on himself through shame, blame, and constant self-criticism. As he says,

> I am as bad as they were. I just ran off and left my mother and sisters to be raped and killed by the soldiers. I am no better. I should be made to admit my crimes and pay for them. I would be willing to do anything to bring them back.

As is evident here, identifying with the aggressor is painful for Vladamir, but it in turn protects against the rage, loss, and grief of losing his family.

Projective identification is another interpersonal defense that requires two people to make it work. One person must unconsciously project a feeling out into the environment. Another person then unconsciously identifies with it and acts it out.

In normal development, projective identification is a tool the child uses to learn how to modulate feelings (Schore, 1994). The child projects feelings, such as sadness, fear, anger, onto the mother. The mother experiences the feeling, identifies it with words, and gives it back to the child in a calmer form.

This same process takes place with people who have unprocessed emotional experience, such as trauma survivors. Clients unconsciously project feelings they don't want to experience into their interactions with others. Often, these people then feel some vague sense of a feeling that is or is not theirs. If the feeling is not labeled, then the family member, friend, or therapist will unconsciously act it out for the survivor.

For example, Andrea cannot feel her rage at the boys who raped her. Instead she feels the shame and the self-hate. So, whenever she is talking to someone, they will feel the anger she cannot experience. They may become enraged at the boys or men in general for her. Sometimes they will act it out toward her by turning on her and saying things like "if you hadn't gotten drunk, it wouldn't have happened."

This is of course, not an exhaustive list of primitive defenses. Higher order defenses such as rationalization, intellectualization, and undoing are also used by trauma survivors, but are not discussed here.

DISTORTED OBJECT RELATIONS

When trauma occurs, the mental representations of self and other become narrowed and limited to that of victim, perpetrator, and abandoning authority for survival. While this internalization is an accurate representation of relationship at the time of trauma, these trauma-based perceptions often become generalized in life. Transferences from the past overlay interpersonal relationships in the present causing confusion, distress, and, ultimately, the acting out of projections.

Transference

Like projective identification, transference is a normal psychological process of development. It is an interpersonal process where the child transfers images of self onto others to discriminate, separate, and create boundaries. As they are reflected back, s/he introjects them into self-organization.

With trauma survivors, transference happens unconsciously, in an effort to sort out the past from the present. Overlays of past relationships shadow present interactions. Many people find themselves in destructive relationships over and over again, in an effort to work through the past, in repetition compulsions.

When Tricia started therapy, she had already been married and divorced twice. She made two suicide attempts when these marriages broke up due to her sexual acting out. She was then married to her third husband, which she stated was a healthy, monogamous marriage. Even in a stable, committed relationship, however, Tricia found herself seeing her husband as her father, who had sexually abused her. This is how she described a typical interaction with her husband:

> Bill and I would go out to dinner together. We would be getting along, laughing, having fun, and then all of a sudden I would get upset. It might be that his hand grazed my bottom when I wasn't expecting it. It could be that he looked at me critically, or his voice tone changed toward me. Immediately, I would feel like I was back at one of the fancy restaurants my father took me to as a little girl. I would be paralyzed and our good evening would be ruined once again.

Whereas transference causes distorted object relations that affect intimate relationships, self-perception is often shaky as well.

EGO STATE CHANGES

Uncontrolled regression, where an emotion triggers an involuntarily shift from one ego state to another, is probably the most disruptive trauma symptom there is. Sometimes these ego state changes are only obvious to the trauma survivor in internal awareness. Clients report they can feel "younger feelings" or hear a "little voice inside." Other times, clients can regress and even look like a 5-year-old child, in a moment's notice.

Vladamir described ego state shifts as part of his daily experience of posttraumatic stress disorder. He reported staying calm at work, but when he got home he would experience uncontrolled rages, and regressions to a preverbal state.

Along with ego state shifts comes the compulsive, unconscious acting out of unprocessed trauma material (Terr, 1991). Researchers and clinicians agree that reenactment is an adaptive response. The unprocessed material is trying to gain entrance to conscious awareness to find words for the experiences. Like all problems with distorted object relations, however, this symptom can result in confusion, projection, and great distress when relating to others.

Tricia was particularly bothered when she would find herself relating to her client as though he were her godfather, who had sadistically abused her for many years. She became fearful, and tried repeatedly to placate this man in the present whenever his voice tone would begin to sound hostile to her.

CHANGES IN SPIRITUALITY

One of the more often overlooked symptoms of violence is its impact on people's spirituality (Culbertson, 2001). For many trauma survivors, trauma brings such a powerful experience of hopelessness, that any belief in a higher power, a god, a force beyond oneself that is good, is destroyed. "Where were you, God?" is a familiar refrain.

In some cases of religious persecution or abuse by the clergy, people are directly traumatized by religion and the people who are its leaders. Cult abuse takes religious practices and distorts them for the sake of power and control. Life, as stated earlier, is profoundly affected by trauma at all levels of basic human functioning.

TRAUMA BUBBLES: A CLIENT-FRIENDLY IMAGE OF TRAUMA

The image and concept of "trauma bubbles" was developed in practice with clients with PTSD to further help them understand the impacts described above. The idea takes the theoretical and experiential information above and puts it in a few simple words, for quick communication between therapist and client. Figure 1.1 shows the elements of a trauma bubble.

Trauma bubbles are encapsulated spheres of active psychological awareness that contain unprocessed experiences. These experiences are dissociated and split off from conscious awareness. Like bubbles, they can be popped unexpectedly, pouring images, sensations, sounds, smells, and tastes into awareness without words.

Trauma bubbles make sense to trauma survivors almost immediately. This graphic image helps clients understand the systematic changes that occur in conscious awareness due to the impact of severe trauma. It can become a shorthand to symbolize the myriad of symptoms that this chapter has presented.

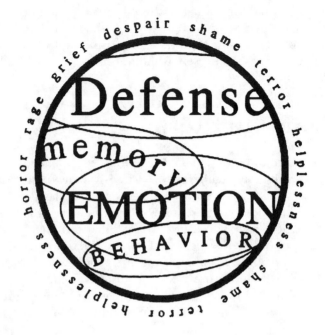

FIGURE 1.1   Trauma bubble.

Andrea immediately embraced the image of trauma bubbles and was able to describe the sexual assault with help from this tool. She said,

> In one bubble is the image of the first boy's face . . . full of rage. In another bubble there are images of many hands grabbing at me. In yet a third I can see myself lying on the floor afterward, alone and paralyzed. And in a fourth bubble, I can feel the edge of terror.

CONCLUSIONS

There are three resounding conclusions that come from presenting this theoretical foundation on trauma:

1. Trauma treatment must address the whole person: body, mind, emotion, and spirit.
2. The core trauma experience needs to be accessed, expressed, and processed for full symptom remission.

3. Talk therapy cannot access unprocessed material stored in the emotional centers of the right brain.

Bessel van der Kolk was the keynote speaker at the 1997 American Society of Group Psychotherapy and Psychodrama. He stated that body-centered, experiential methods are the "treatment of choice" for traumatized people. Chapter 2 now explains why that is true.

CHAPTER TWO

Experiential Therapy with Trauma Survivors

> Experiential therapy is not another school, another method, but a meta-orientation, a certain way of using various vocabularies, theories, and procedures. Experiential therapy focuses on being rather than talking about; on the on-going, lived present flow of experience. . . . But before there was an experiential therapy there was the experiential in therapy. It has always been there in good therapy.
>
> —(Friedman, 1976, p. 236)

CHAPTER OVERVIEW

As illustrated in chapter 1, trauma impacts human functioning at every level of development. Overwhelming experience causes changes in cognition and emotion, developmental delays, and loss of connection, hope, and spirit. Experiential therapy is suggested as the treatment of choice as it treats body, mind, emotions, behaviors and spirit from a client-centered approach.

Chapter 2 presents the theory and research on experiential therapy with PTSD. Classical psychodrama is demonstrated as the seminal action method and a foundation of the Therapeutic Spiral Model. Clients continue to bring this material alive to show a match between nonverbal trauma symptoms and experiential therapy as a treatment of choice. As van der Kolk (1996b) stated,

> Prone to action, and deficient in words, these patients (trauma survivors) can often express their internal states more articulately in physical movements or in pictures than in words. Utilizing drawings and *psychodrama* may help

them develop a language that is essential for effective communication and for the symbolic transformation that can occur in psychotherapy. (p. 195, emphasis added)

GENERAL OVERVIEW

Until the publication of the 4th edition of the *Handbook of Psychotherapy and Behavior Change* (Bergin & Garfield, 1994a), experiential psychotherapy had received little academic notice or research support. Even solid systems of psychotherapy, such as focusing, Gestalt therapy, and psychodrama, were relegated to "fringe therapies" due to lack of theoretical understanding and research findings. Researchers that contributed to that edition, however, demonstrated that experiential psychotherapy is equally as effective as psychodynamic, behavioral, and cognitive-behavioral therapies (Greenberg, Elliott, & Lietaer, 1994). In fact, studies show that it is *experiential processes* that produce change across all theoretical orientations. Active experiencing and adaptive use of emotion are the core principles of change in experiential psychotherapy. They are key to all good therapy hours (Greenberg & Van Balen, 1998).

Clients have long proclaimed the effectiveness and depth of healing with experiential methods. As Jim put it,

> I had talked myself blue in the face at meetings, group sessions, and individual work with my addictions counselor. I was sober, but I wasn't happy. Words just never reached those images, sensations, and feelings that I tried to blot out.
>
> When I found action methods in inpatient treatment, I thought "this is it!" Here was a place that I could tell what was happening to me—without words. We used drawings, movement, and psychodrama. I finally found relief from the flashbacks and nightmares and for that I am forever grateful.

Today, we have an agreed upon definition of what makes a therapy experiential, as well as research to support it's use with trauma related diagnoses (Greenberg, Watson, & Lietaer, 1998).

DEFINITION OF EXPERIENTIAL PSYCHOTHERAPY

> Experiential therapies all define the facilitation of experiencing as the key therapeutic task, and almost all view the therapeutic relationship as potentially curative. Experiential approaches emphasize the importance of active, process-directive intervention procedures oriented toward deepening experience

within the context of a person-centered relationship. (Greenberg, Elliott, & Lietaer, 1994, pp. 509–510)

Remember that research on the neurobiology of trauma demonstrated that unprocessed trauma material is stored in the right brain as sensori-motor representations—fragmented images, smells, sensations, nonverbal behavior, and emotional nuances—without cognitive labels. Action methods directly access these places without words, so they can be experienced, expressed, and integrated into new personal narratives of healing.

Experiential therapy increases treatment effectiveness with symptoms such as flashbacks, body memories, dissociated affects, primitive defenses, and ego state changes. As Turner, McFarlane, and van der Kolk (1996) state, the focus of treatment needs to be

> . . . on helping the individual to process and come to terms with the horrifying, overwhelming *experience* of trauma. The importance of capturing the experience in its *full range of representations* goes beyond the person's simply remembering and reporting the verbal schemata. Treatment must address the somatosensory, emotional, biological, as well as, cognitive dimensions of experience. (p. 546, emphasis added)

Andrea found that her participation in an experiential workshop enabled her to deal with her anorexia more thoroughly than talk therapy alone. In her words,

> I never wanted to see or feel my body again when I started therapy. Talk therapy let me "talk around" my body. I could talk about body image, weighing myself over and over again, and how I never felt hungry. It wasn't hard to figure out *why* I felt like that about myself . . . but ya know, that didn't change anything.
>
> During one weekend TSM workshop, that all changed. I was asked to role reverse and become my "body double" and speak to myself from that role [active experiencing]. I just started crying and crying, saying, "I want to live again" [adaptive affect], and, "I feel like I am dead. Please let me out of here" [regression in the service of the ego]. From then on, I couldn't ignore my body anymore.

EXPERIENTIAL PRINCIPLES OF CHANGE

In the clinical description above, the three principles of change that are core to experiential methods were aptly demonstrated:

- Active experiencing
- Adaptive use of affect
- Regression in the service of the ego

When working with trauma survivors, these same principles are crucial to success with the dissociated, nonverbal symptoms of PTSD.

ACTIVE EXPERIENCING

Gendlin (1962), an experiential therapist and researcher, operationalized the process of "active experiencing" as a necessary ingredient in all successful psychotherapy. Active experiencing, which he called focusing (1996), is an attentional skill that brings unconscious and automatic sensations, perceptions, nonverbal behaviors, emotional nuances and impulses, into conscious awareness, so they can be experienced and further processed.

Clients who are working on unprocessed trauma material and dissociated affects often live in a state of uncontrolled reexperiencing of the fragments of their traumas. Active experiencing is not a choice, but a violent repeat of the past. Teaching trauma survivors how to consciously choose to actively experience the flashbacks and body memories gives them an immediate power over some of the most disturbing PTSD symptoms.

Process directive interventions by an experiential therapist teach how to focus on and change internal perceptions related to past trauma. Feelings are identified and expressed by choice in safe and appropriate settings. Clients gain a sense of control and choice early in experiential psychotherapy.

Tricia learned how to focus on the flashbacks that were interrupting her work. She found this skill gave her back a sense of control in her daily life. She said,

> I thought I was going crazy when the flashbacks first started. I would be in the library at the firm or at home. All of a sudden I would feel bombarded by images and feelings from my past. I knew they were from the past. I remembered the physical and sexual violence in my family. I just didn't see why this was happening to me now.
>
> In therapy, I learned how to—if not embrace these flashbacks and body memories—at least how to not crumble when they intruded. I found I could let them come into my mind, notice them, and write them down. Then I

could choose to process them later in therapy. I felt back in control again. I could go to work and not be scared I was gonna become a "little girl" in the middle of a meeting.

USE OF ADAPTIVE AFFECT

Emotions communicate valuable information about safety, individual needs, and connection to others (Greenberg, Korman, & Pavio, 2001). There are two components to any emotion: experiencing it and expressing it. For every emotion, the mind actively experiences and organizes the complex network of sensations, nonverbal behaviors, intuitive nuances, and energetic connections that make up each primary affect—joy, anger, grief, surprise, disgust, et cetera (Greenberg, 2001). In turn, these emotions provide valuable information about the self, others, and the world.

Trauma survivors, however, automatically cut off their emotions at the time of trauma as part of survival. In fact, for many people, expressing feelings would have made the violence worse or even resulted in death. As a result of such traumatic learning, many trauma survivors deny, dissociate, and project their feelings so automatically they often have no idea what a healthy emotion actually feels like. Their only experience of emotion is the unpredictable intensity of dissociated rage, terror, despair, or hatred when a trauma bubble explodes. To learn how to identify, experience, and adaptively express these dissociated feelings safely is a core component of change for trauma survivors (Cornell & Olio, 1991; Kellermann, 2000).

As a counselor at a refugee agency in Sydney, Vladamir told himself that he should be able to control his own emotions when working with the newer refugees just getting resettled. When he would go home from a day of listening to new people recently torn from their families, however, he was unable to control his own emotional outbursts. He said,

I came home the other night from work. It had been a long day. A new family came in . . . from Montenegro . . . a place that was supposed to still be safe. I found them temporary housing and heard how the war continues. The mother had lost her son. I was devastated. I could barely stay in the room while they shared their sorrows.

When I got home I punched the wall. I just couldn't help myself. I was so angry, so enraged at what people do to each other. Each day I do my best to help people . . . to do what is right . . . but the reality is I am so angry I could kill. God help me.

A few months later, Vladamir participated in his second weekend of experiential training at the refugee center. As part of a drama, he was able to express his "murderous rage" at a set of auxiliaries who took the role of the soldiers. At the end of his training course he stated the following:

> One of the most important moments for me in this training was when I was able to finally express my own rage. There in a group of professional colleagues, which included two women who were former refugees from Bosnia . . . I was able to pound my fists, shout at God, and share my pain. To me, that is what made the difference in my own healing.

Experiential therapy values the use of adaptive affect and provides structured steps to safely express dissociated emotions for trauma survivors. Classical psychodrama has many ways to express feelings. People beat chairs with foam batacas. They throw punches at punching bags. They scream out the rage that has been held in for years. Despair is met with holding and the space to fully cry for the losses and grief of traumatic experiences. Pain is witnessed with compassion and healing. Dances of joy and joining of spirits all happen in psychodrama as an experiential method of group psychotherapy.

REGRESSION IN THE SERVICE OF THE EGO

Slavson (1951) stated that the true value of catharsis is that it produces therapeutic regression in the service of the ego. The reason that conscious regression does repair the ego is based on state dependent learning. Each state has its own experiential learning history and must be accessed directly to be experienced and processed for change to occur.

Experiential psychotherapy directly addresses different ego states so they can be fully explored and integrated. In this way, symptoms such as body memories and flashbacks are fully healed, not just managed. As Zerka Moreno (personal communication, June 20, 2001) observed, psychodrama brings the past into the present where it is safe to consciously reexperience it. When properly structured, regression in the service of the ego can access unprocessed trauma material encoded in state dependent learning. This is crucial in order for trauma survivors to reach full developmental repair.

Tricia used the principle of regression in the service of the ego quite well. Early on in therapy, she was singularly focused on the question,

"Why is this happening to me now?" Her lawyer's mind wanted to understand the logical link between past and present. She couldn't let go of her obsession on "why now?"—so, we contracted for a drama that would find and label these links through conscious regression and active experiencing of her past.

Director: You say you can "see" the scene of your godfather throwing you against the wall? This is the memory that keeps intruding on you in the law library?

Tricia: Yes, over and over and over again. I just cannot make it stop sometimes. Other times, I can write it down and know I can look at it later. But today . . . it just wouldn't stop and I got almost no work done.

Director: Will you reverse roles with that little girl who is being thrown against the wall? You can take your curiosity with you and see what you have to say from that small victim place.

Tricia in child role: I can't make him stop. I am too little. I can't do it. Help me! Help me! Something bad is gonna happen. Oh no, I'm really scared. Help me!

Director: Who are you talking to, Tricia? Someone in the past? Someone in the present?

Tricia in child role: I am talking to my mother. I want my mama to take care of me. I don't want to have to make it stop. I want her to do that for me!

Director: Reverse roles into your observing ego role.

Tricia in an observing ego role: I guess in the present, I'd be talking to myself, the part of me that has abandoned ship since the chaos showed up. It's like I need to talk to the adult part of me and get things back into control.

RESEARCH

The *Handbook of Experiential Psychotherapy*, edited by Greenberg, Watson, and Lietaer (1998, In Press), documents treatment effectiveness of experiential therapy with a range of clinical disorders that are relevant to treating trauma:

- Depression (Greenberg, Watson, & Goldman, 1998);
- Anxiety disorders (Wolfe & Sigl, 1998);

- Borderline personality disorder (Eckert & Biermann-Ratjen, 1998);
- Posttraumatic stress disorder (Elliott, Davis, & Slatick, 1998; Elliott, Suter, et al., 1996).

Experiential therapy has been shown to be as effective as psychodynamic and cognitive behavioral therapy for a wide range of problems, and is emerging as the treatment of choice for many practitioners working with PTSD.

Psychodrama was developed in practice with trauma survivors of earlier generations—World War I and II refugees, prostitutes, and patients no one else could treat. It provides theoretical constructs and action techniques to guide experiential treatment (Blatner, 1997; Hug, 1997). Psychodrama will now be discussed in greater detail.

CLASSICAL PSYCHODRAMA: THE SEMINAL ACTION METHOD WITH TRAUMA

Classical psychodrama was developed by J. L. Moreno (1947, 1953, 1973), together with his wife and colleague, Zerka T. Moreno (1969). Psychodrama is a method of healing both personal and collective trauma that incorporates the transpersonal, interpersonal, and intrapsychic areas of life. It is the prototypical experiential method of healing and has been applied in many communities in the world for the past 75 years (Blatner, 1997).

DEFINITION

As a method of experiential group psychotherapy, psychodrama is a complex system. It has been defined and refined over the years, though, until now we have a basic agreement of what constitutes psychodrama (Dayton, 1994; Kipper, 1997). The basic structure of a psychodrama session is comprised of warm-up, action, and sharing (Goldman & Morrison, 1984; Hollander, 1969). The group warms up to a theme. A protagonist is chosen and puts a story into action. People share their own experiences of the drama. They connect it to their past to learn something new about their future.

Psychodrama, by definition (Kellermann, 1992) includes a minimum of one scene that uses role-playing methods. Basic techniques include spontaneity training, double, mirror, role training, role reversal, soliloquy, aside, and future projection.

There are many excellent books, chapters, and articles on the original formulations of psychodrama (Blatner, 1995, 1996, 2000; Buchanan, 1980; Haworth, 1998; Holmes, 1991; Leveton, 1977/1992). Recent volumes detail applications to business, clinical practice, legal and political structures, and large organizations (Fox, 1987; Holmes & Karp, 1991; Holmes, Karp, & Watson, 1994; Hudgins & Kipper, 1998; Karp, Holmes, & Tauvon, 1998; Kellermann & Hudgins, 2000). These references are rich in client stories, anecdotal evidence, and qualitative research (Wilkins, 1997).

In her fifth month, Andrea wanted to do a future projection. She wanted to see what it would be like to be rid of PTSD and be open to young men again. She set up a single scene where she picked people to play the roles she said she needed. Tricia was her "bright mind." Susan played her "shining star." Michael had a great time playing "healthy sexuality." Vladamir became an "open and knowing heart." With these roles in place, Andrea enacted meeting a man at an art show she was going to with her parents in 3 months. At the end of the future projection, she said, "Maybe I'm more ready than I thought. I had a good time!"

THE CONSTRUCT OF SURPLUS REALITY

All psychodramatic techniques have the goal of making the client's internal reality overtly visible both to self and others (Moreno, Blomkvist, & Rützel, 2000). That is, psychodramatic techniques concretize and tangibly present all aspects of the client's internal experience, both verbal and nonverbal, for the purpose of increased awareness, exploration, and change.

According to Moreno (1965),

> Psychodrama consists not merely of the enactment of episodes, past, present, and future, which are experienced and conceivable within the framework of reality. There is in psychodrama a mode of experiencing, which goes beyond reality, which provides the subject with a new and more extensive experience of reality, a surplus reality. Surplus reality is not a loss but an enrichment of reality. The expansion of experience is made possible by methods not used in life—auxiliary egos, auxiliary chair, double, role reversal, mirror . . . and others. (pp. 212–213)

It was surplus reality that really made a difference in Jim's healing. He said,

> One of the best things about psychodrama is that you get to do things that you always wanted to happen but they never did. One time, I had someone play my grandfather—my mother's father. He was a great old man. He would sit on the porch and play his harmonica and watch us kids play baseball. In the drama, I got to sit next to him and talk to him again. This time I talked about everything I had never told him as a kid.
>
> I told him about Dad beating me. I told him how scared I had been. I even told him how scared I was now . . . how those beatings seemed somehow to still be happening to me in my mind, and in my body, each and everyday.
>
> The group member playing my grandpa said, "Jimmy, Jimmy . . . I am so sorry that happened to you. I knew something wasn't right in your family, but your mother she would never tell me a thing when I asked . . . just told me it was none of my business. I'm glad you are telling me now. Sit here, sit down next to me on the old porch . . . and tell me how you are now."
>
> I did tell him everything . . . the violence, the terror, the hatred, the guns, the belts, the nightsticks. He touched my face. At that point I cried like a baby and my old grandpa patted me on the shoulder, let me rest against his heart, and told me what a good man I had become.

SPONTANEITY THEORY

The goal of all psychodrama methods is to access the experience of spontaneity in order to produce creative and new solutions to old problems (Kipper, 2000). Moreno (1947/1973) described spontaneity as an unconservable, renewable energy source that is overtly detectable in how an individual warms up to—becomes conscious of—a given situation. In 1920, Moreno boldly stated spontaneity comes from the "god within" and made spirituality a central focus of his healing methods.

When trauma happens, no amount of personal spontaneity, creativity, or belief in God is able to prevent overwhelming horror, pain, and grief from happening. Survival is all that matters. In the case of trauma survivors, an emphasis both on spontaneity and spirituality provides an antidote to the helplessness and despair of many trauma experiences. During a session to build spontaneity, Andrea said, "I want to be a guardian angel to myself." The group then psychodramatically dressed her in angel garb—white, gold-tipped wings; stars for a halo; a soft flowing iridescent aqua gown; a healing wand; jewels around her neck;

flowers in her hair; and golden light flowing from her fingertips. This surplus reality experience of "something greater than herself" helped Andrea's self-esteem more in one night than years of standard talk therapy could ever do.

ROLE THEORY

Role theory, another central tenet of psychodrama, provides a useful framework for trauma survivors because it joins cognitive, affective, and behavioral states together for easy categorization (Buchanan, 1984). Moreno (1961) said that the self is made up of the roles we play. Psychodrama utilizes the concept of role to bridge the theatrical and the therapeutic elements of healing (Blatner, 1991). It is also useful with cultural perspectives (Clayton, 1994; Tomasulo, 2000).

Role theory provides an understandable structure for object relations when working with trauma survivors (Holmes, 1992). It connects medical diagnosis and the client's experience of self. Roles demystify psychiatric labels such as multiple personality and dissociative identity disorder, a boon to people who have experienced severe trauma. It normalizes the experience of split parts of self, so clients can access information in trauma bubbles without shame.

One of the clinical action structures in the Therapeutic Spiral Model, the trauma survivor's intrapsychic role atom (Cossa & Hudgins, 1998; Toscani & Hudgins, 1996), details the prescriptive, trauma-based, and transformative roles that are internalized from the impact and healing of trauma. Tricia used this role template to create a healing experience for herself:

> In one of my final sessions at a workshop, I looked around at all the parts of myself on the stage. I had a wise woman, a guardian angel, my best friend, my dog, my serenity, and my trust in others. These roles were all there to support me now. They held the wounded child, the rage queen, and the controlled robot with compassion and love. I felt I was seeing myself . . . my whole self for the first time. And ya know . . . I think I'm pretty special!

RESEARCH

For many years, classical psychodrama was acclaimed by clients but had little research support. In the last 10 years that has changed, and now there is a body of empirical research that includes over 100 studies (M. Wieser, personal communication, May 22, 2001). Current reports summarize treatment effectiveness in a wide range of applications. Specific studies and case presentations show the successful use of psychodrama with many trauma related diagnoses:

- Addiction (Dayton, 2000a,b; Forst, 2001; Fuhlrodt, 1990; Rustin & Olson, 1993);
- Borderline personality disorder (Sidorsky, 1984);
- Depression (Dogner & Valip, 1994; Farmer, 1998; Mehdi, Sen, & Sen, 1997; Rezaeian, Mazumdar, & Sen, 1997);
- Domestic violence (Burger, 1994);
- Dissociative identity disorder (Altman, 2000, 1993; Leutz, 2000; Raaz, Carlson-Sabelli, & Sabelli, 1993; Reynolds, 1996);
- Eating disorders (Baratka, 1994; Hudgins, 1989; Widlake, 1997);
- High risk adolescents and families (Bannister & Huntington, 2002; Chimera, C., 2002; Cossa, 2002);
- PTSD (Baumgartner, 1986; Burge, 1996; Carbonell & Parteleno-Barehmi, 1999; Hudgins & Drucker, 1998; Hudgins, Drucker, & Metcalf, 2000; Ragsdale, Cox, Finn, & Eisler, 1996);
- Sexual abuse (Bannister, 1990, 1991, 1997, 2000; Carbonell & Parteleno-Barehmi, 1999; Hudgins, 1998, 2000; Karp, 1991);
- Sex offenders (Baim, 2000; Robson, 2000);
- Somatization disorder (Kellermann, 1996).

Research on the Therapeutic Spiral Model

The next chapter introduces the Therapeutic Spiral Model (TSM) more fully. Prior antecedents to the Therapeutic Spiral Model can be found in earlier attempts to structure psychodramatic treatment with clients who have experienced trauma (Altman, 1992, 1993; Bannister, 1991, 1997; Dayton, 1997; Hudgins, 1989, 1998).

The Three-Child Model of recovery (Sheridan & Hudgins, 1990) was the seed of the present intrapsychic role atom in the Therapeutic Spiral Model. It initially detailed the sleeping-child, the wounded-child, and the adult-child roles to describe the internalized representations of growing up in an alcoholic home. These roles have been expanded to create the trauma survivor's intrapsychic role atom in TSM (Toscani & Hudgins, 1996).

A single case research design showed that the containing double, a TSM manualized intervention module, significantly decreased dissociation and general trauma symptoms for a woman with PTSD from childhood sexual abuse (Hudgins & Drucker, 1998; Hudgins, Drucker, & Metcalf, 2000). Currently, we are beginning a cross-cultural project testing this same intervention in clients diagnosed with PTSD from a variety of stressors in Australia, Canada, South Africa, the United Kingdom, and the United States.

CONCLUSIONS

Despite research evidence and client acclaim, many therapists still fear using experiential methods with trauma survivors. Action methods can directly access unprocessed trauma material and intense dissociated feelings—this is both the good news and the bad. It is good news because developmental repair can happen. It is problematic because all experiential methods can increase the risk for uncontrolled regression and retraumatization in the hands of untrained, unskilled, or overzealous practitioners.

Many people have trained and become certified by the American Board of Examiners (1982), the British Psychodrama Association (1993), the Australian and New Zealand Psychodrama Association (1989), and other boards around the world. (See Appendix B for information and websites.) Certification follows a rigorous postgraduate training program with direct supervision and practice to promote competent and safe use of psychodrama, sociometry, and group psychotherapy.

What the Therapeutic Spiral Model adds to classical psychodrama is additional focus on directing trauma-based scenes from a clinical perspective. According to the work of Zerka Moreno (1959, 1965), psychodrama is often seen as a method of catharsis and emotional release, but it is also a method of containment and integration. TSM carries that one step further by developing clinical action structures to guide the use of action methods to increase safety when treating trauma survivors.

There are four main differences between the practice of classical psychodrama and the Therapeutic Spiral Model:

1) TSM focuses on change in internal self-organization and internalization of trauma-based roles. Classical psychodrama focuses on change in interpersonal relationships.

2)   TSM works from a clinical foundation about how trauma affects people. All directing decisions are made as clinical decisions, not dramatic ones.

3)   An action trauma team is needed to provide safety for the full depth of conscious reexperiencing that can be achieved with experiential methods. TSM assumes that projective identification is an active defense in all groups of trauma survivors. This greatly affects group treatment as will be evident in the chapters ahead.

4)   The unique clinical action structures of TSM create a balance between active experiencing, emotional expression, and narrative labeling to achieve full developmental repair through regression in the service of the ego.

The Therapeutic Spiral Model embraces the theory and methods of classical psychodrama. Its contribution is to make experiential therapy safer for trauma survivors.

CHAPTER THREE

The Therapeutic Spiral Model: Visual Images and Clinical Structures

CHAPTER OVERVIEW

Chapter 2 showed that experiential methods are powerful tools of change when working with trauma (Elliott et al., 1998). Spontaneity and role theories, foundations of psychodrama, were used to explain the impact of trauma in easily understood terms. The Therapeutic Spiral Model (TSM) was prescribed as a treatment of choice for trauma survivors as it combines the best of experiential methods and clinical expertise.

This chapter introduces the "clinical action structures" that modify classical psychodramatic methods in the TSM. These clinical action structures provide a structured set of action experiences designed to achieve a clinical goal: containment, conscious re-experiencing, meaning making, et cetera. These are TSM structures that utilize action techniques, guided from a clinician's perspective.

This chapter introduces the first clinical action structure: the spiral image. A series of six TSM clinical action structures are described that were designed to meet two initial clinical goals with trauma survivors:

- to create a safe container for increased experiencing, and
- to quickly support the emergence of new narrative meanings.

THE SPIRAL IMAGE

To begin, imagine a visual image of a spiral—shaped like a DNA model with three interwoven strands. Each strand is a different color. Purple

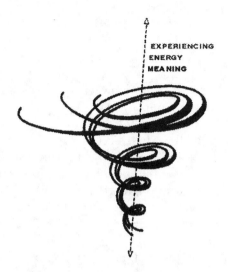

EXPERIENCING
ENERGY
MEANING

FIGURE 3.1   The healthy spiral.

is for energy. Teal symbolizes experiencing. Rose is the color designated for new meaning. The colors course up and down the spiral in various shades, intensities, and rhythms.

This spiral image is introduced to help communication between therapist and client, when words are in short supply. In this case, the spiral provides narrative labeling of strengths and disrupted self-organization at an early point in trauma work. This quick simplification of complex emotional states helps facilitate those difficult moments when trauma symptoms threaten to take over therapeutic interventions. Because it is a visual image the spiral can be used to bridge the gap between experiences of trauma and the words to describe their impact. It can also be used as a clinical guide for early interventions in TSM.

HISTORY OF THE SPIRAL

There are three reasons that I chose the spiral image to represent this innovative method of clinical experiential therapy with trauma survivors. Each one helps people identify with the image and learn to use it to begin to put words to traumas that remain unprocessed in trauma bubbles.

Clients often describe their experience of trauma with images like "worlds colliding" and "black holes." They use metaphors that embody images that are unpredictable, out of control, and destructive. The images and intense feelings of trauma can haunt people long after trauma has happened.

Andrea shared that no matter how hard she tried to push the images and feelings out of her mind by counting, weighing, and exercising, the faces of the boys who raped her kept intruding on her in the present. When this happened she would become overwhelmed with terror or rage. She said she felt like she would get hit by a tornado.

The image of a spiral, a therapeutic spiral, gives trauma survivors an alternative perception to the experience of chaos. A quick call to go "up the spiral" can signal a change needed in the clinical direction of the session, when the nonverbal symptoms of PTSD threaten to take over cognitive resources.

Andrea quickly used the therapeutic spiral image to learn to call for help when she was triggered during an experiential session. She would say, "more energy, I'm getting lost" and I would suggest intervention modules of containment or spontaneity. "How could this happen?" would initiate methods that facilitate cognitive processing.

Another reason that I use the spiral image is to symbolize the focus on spirituality that is core to the Therapeutic Spiral Model. As our teams met indigenous people over the past 10 years—Native Americans; Australian Aborigines; Celtic Irish; New Zealand Maori; South Pacific Islanders; African, South American, and Korean shamans—we saw the spiral incorporated into many symbols of healing around the world. In Western medicine, the physician's staff, the caduceus with its entwined snakes, resembles a spiral and means, "do no harm."

In many cases, traumatic experience is caused by humans. In all cases, overwhelming catastrophe is beyond the human capacity to cope. Thus, it is my core belief that trauma survivors need to make sense of what happened to them in a way that is beyond individual experiences. I choose to call this experience spiritual, in the Therapeutic Spiral Model.

The third reason I chose the spiral images connects psychodrama into earlier clinical structures. In classical psychodrama, the development of the experiential action goes from "the periphery to the center" in what has been called a psychodramatic spiral (Goldman & Morrison, 1984). Enactment proceeds from assessment scenes in the present life of the protagonist and "spirals" into connected scenes from the past. Unique to the Therapeutic Spiral Model are these specific clinical action structures that prescribe a set of structured action experiences to reach a clinical goal.

A CLINICAL ACTION STRUCTURE

The spiral image and structure maintain the balance of thinking and feeling that is crucial to the use of all action methods with trauma survivors. There are six action experiences that are presented to build energy, increase experiencing, and increase meaning making.

THE THERAPEUTIC SPIRAL

The therapeutic spiral is a visual image to help bridge the gap between active experiencing of trauma bubbles and the narrative labeling needed to complete cognitive processing. As a first intervention, unprocessed and disruptive sensorimotor experiences can be understood in the simple terms of the three strands of the spiral: energy, experiencing, and meaning.

This initial division provides a simple order to the chaos of fragmented trauma perceptions, thoughts, feelings, and the primitive defenses that follow them. For just a moment, all experience can be labeled simply: Energy—helpful or not? Experiencing—too much, not enough? Meaning—does it make sense or are you overwhelmed? With these questions answered, the therapist can guide the process into a positive, upwardly spiraling direction of attention and focus.

Tricia used the concept of the therapeutic spiral image almost immediately to understand her experience of flashbacks—"being sucked into the spirals of the past, while stuck in the present." We worked to discriminate between the experience of the pull of the past and the choice to instead focus on the here and now. This allowed her to learn to "spiral up out of the chaos," giving interventions direction and purpose in easy words.

THE TRAUMA SPIRAL

When trauma hits, the spiral map is frozen in time. The strands of energy, experiencing, and meaning do not interact or blend. Instead, they become fixed, crushed by the trauma. Conscious movement up and down the spiral becomes stuck, chaotic, and unpredictable. The

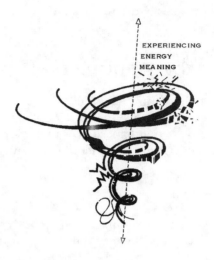

FIGURE 3.2   The trauma spiral.

image of the trauma spiral shows the uncontrolled energy. Experiencing becomes constricted or explosive and dangerous. Personal narratives are not connected to what really happened in life, and so provide poor guides for the future.

As with the construct of trauma bubbles, most survivors find that these two spiral images immediately help them identify and express their internal experiences of trauma more clearly. Simply put, you can ask someone, "Are you in a therapeutic spiral or a trauma spiral right now?" When answered, this question begins to provide a container of understanding for many of the confusing symptoms of PTSD.

Andrea found that she could say, "Too much . . . move to meaning," when she started to feel overwhelmed with her feelings or when she felt she was starting to get dissociated. She could find the therapeutic spiral image when she started to get triggered into terror—a place that was without words.

GUIDING THE SPIRAL: SIX ACTION EXPERIENCES

ENERGY: BUILDING A STATE OF SPONTANEOUS LEARNING

The first strand of the spiral image is called energy. Energy provides the fuel for life and healing in the Therapeutic Spiral Model. Energy is embodied in a sense of physical vitality and aliveness. It connects humans to each other and to something greater than self. It can create universal and lasting meaning from personal catastrophe.

The Therapeutic Spiral Model defines energy as the experience of a state of spontaneous learning where new solutions are possible to old trauma patterns (E. Yorke, personal communication, Sept. 15, 1997). The goal of all interventions in TSM is to establish and maintain this healing state. The Therapeutic Spiral Model operationalizes the state of spontaneous learning through the identification and enactment of a set of prescriptive roles. Prescriptive roles are needed for healthy functioning to achieve observation, restoration, and containment with symptoms of PTSD (see chapter 5). When these roles are developed, the first clinical action structure is completed.

Concretizing the Observing Ego (OE) Role

The first role that is concretized is that of the observing ego. The team creates an action experience that increases awareness of the part of self that can neutrally observe and self reflect what is happening during trauma work. It can be externalized in any number of ways.

Most often, TSM workshops start off with participants choosing a card, poem, object, etc., to "be their witness role." Then they discuss the role with at least one other person to increase group connections. The card or object is then placed somewhere in the room to mark a physical space to hold the role of observation for each person. The first clinical objective is met. The ability to observe self and make choices is established prior to any further action structures.

Restorative Roles: The Circle of Scarves

The second clinical objective is to increase roles of restoration and containment, following the OE role. Again, this is the pre-trauma work of the spiral image and helps put psychological boundaries and narrative labels on present experiencing.

The team leader usually structures the physical building of a circle of scarves to be a visual container for the experiential work to be done. She or he will say,

> Pick one or more scarves to represent your strengths. What strengths do you need to do the work you came to do? You can use personal, interpersonal,

and transpersonal strengths to create a safe place where you can find new endings to old memories.

Team members and participants enact strengths, sometimes with a sound and movement, and then place their scarves to form part of the boundary. The circle of scarves creates a physical space that visually shows containment, made up of pretty colors and different textures.

EXPERIENCING: SAFELY CONCRETIZING THE PAST

The second strand in the therapeutic spiral image is called experiencing and is the defining characteristic of all experiential methods of change (Greenberg, Watson, et al., 1998).The second strand of the spiral image focuses on how to consciously reexperience trauma bubbles safely and effectively.

In the TSM, active experiencing of the unprocessed material in trauma bubbles is clinically structured. The action interventions chosen maintain cognitive control of all regressive processes. These action steps are pre-trauma work, most often completed in a group setting.

Spectrograms

A standard action tool for initial assessment is a spectrogram. The team leader or individual therapist creates an imaginary line down the middle of the circle of scarves. People place themselves somewhere on the line with opposite poles marked, to show where they are on a certain criteria. Some examples of questions asked and answered by the use of spectrograms in TSM workshops follow:

1. How many self-care resources have you set up for yourself for the weekend?
2. What is your experience with psychodrama?
3. What is your experience with TSM?
4. Are you feeling OK or distressed right now?
5. What is your comfort level with touch?
6. How easily do you express your feelings?

Action Sociograms

The next clinical action step with a group of trauma survivors is to build connections of trust and safety. The stronger the interpersonal connections among group members, the deeper the level of experiencing that can happen with this support.

Action sociograms are set structures designed to increase group cohesion and provide narrative labeling of the choices in the group (Hale, 1985). The TSM team leader explains how to make a choice and then asks the group to "Put your hand on the shoulder of the person who

- you've known the longest in the room.
- you trust the most right now.
- reminds you of your best friend.
- could take the role of your inner child.
- you have a dual role with in the room, where you are in the dependent role in this relationship—as client; trainee; supervisee; employee."

These questions make overt many of the positive connections in the group. This activity also quickly identifies any issues that may become problematic: dual roles, transferences, projections/projective identifications, etc.

Circle Sociometry

Another action technique used in TSM groups to increase experiencing is circle sociometry (Hale, 1985). It provides an action sequence to increase feelings of inclusion and connection. It also assesses and contains group members' ability to label and share trauma symptoms. The team leader says,

> The team will ask some questions about how trauma has affected you. If you meet the criteria, you step into the circle. If you don't identity, then you stand on the outside of the circle. Different people will step in for different things. After the team has asked some questions, we want you to ask what you need to know to feel safe in this group.

The team starts off with easy questions that don't require much revealing self-disclosure. This teaches the action step of moving in and out of the circle and warms the group up for deeper levels of sharing. For example,

- Who has a pet? Subdivide into dog and cat people.
- Who is married or in a committed partnership?
- Who is the eldest child? Only child? More than five siblings?
- Who has problems with anger? With depression?
- Who has problems with addictions or eating disorders?

Make sure to intersperse strength-building questions among the ones that increase experiencing of trauma material to continue the TSM balance of thinking and feeling. For example,

- Who has been abused in childhood? As an adult?
- Who was physically abused? Sexually abused in the family? Outside the family? Abused by more than one person?
- Who found a good mother that helped as a kid?
- Who had a best friend that made a difference?
- Who has support as an adult?
- Who has been connected to suicide? Others? Your own attempts?
- Who can promise no self-harm tonight?

A good idea is to ask the group what they want to know about each other and encourage them to call out their criteria. If they ask too many trauma-based questions, a team member can control the increased experiencing by asking about a lighter, fun, or even silly criteria, like who has 10 toes?

MEANING: PUT WORDS TO THE UNSPEAKABLE

The third strand of the therapeutic spiral is called meaning. People live their lives based on the personal narrative they have made about past experience and their hopes for the future. When cognitive meanings are attached to accurate experiencing, these symbolic representations create realistic goals and expectations about self and others.

When trauma distorts self-perception and belief systems, however, it is important to spend time sorting out a new narrative based on personal experience. In TSM, this is a thread that runs through all the experiential work that focuses on meaning making.

Use of an Art Project

The final experiential exercise on Friday night at a workshop is to begin an art project that will run through the whole weekend workshop. No matter what the medium (collages, clay models, sand-trays, etc.), these projects always follow the same TSM format based on the spiral image. Art projects provide containment for unconscious trauma material and narrative labeling of its transformation.

Tricia found the use of sand-trays particularly appealing to her. In one workshop, she found judges and fairies and greenery to mark her strengths on Friday night. The next day her sand-tray looked like a cyclone had hit it. She had all the pieces knocked over by her trauma. Furniture was upended. A great big black and red ball sat in the middle of her art project to show how it felt to have body memories and flashbacks disrupting her day-to-day practice as an attorney. On Sunday, the ball of trauma was smaller. Now it was contained behind a fence. Her sand-tray showed a new order.

CONCLUSIONS

Therapists, clients, and most recently researchers are all calling for experiential methods as a faster and more effective way to treat the symptoms people experience from trauma. Classical psychodrama as modified and presented by the Therapeutic Spiral Model is a safe and effective method of treatment for all trauma survivors.

This chapter presented the first TSM clinical action structure, the therapeutic spiral image. It showed how this image can be used to achieve a balance among energy, experiencing, and meaning to promote safety and prevent uncontrolled regression. This is the first step in using experiential methods with trauma survivors to prevent retraumatization. The next section details further clinical action structures for containment and safe, conscious reexperiencing of trauma based roles.

PART TWO

The Unique Clinical Action Structures of TSM

The second section of this book presents three additional clinical action structures that guide practice in the Therapeutic Spiral Model. These are the unique developments that seek to provide containment with experiential methods in TSM. Client stories continue to make the material come alive.

Chapter 4 describes the use of an action trauma team to work with groups of trauma survivors. TSM, in its depth is a team intervention and includes a team leader, an assistant leader, and a trained auxiliary ego. Together these roles provide the maximum support and safety for conscious reexperiencing, as they provide the functions of therapist, analyst, sociometrist, and producer to TSM dramas.

Chapter 5 details the clinical map that guides all experiential interventions when working with PTSD. The trauma survivors intrapsychic role atom prescribes roles of restoration, observation, and containment as pre-trauma work. Trauma-based roles that are internalized by overwhelming experiences can be explored with the additional support and safety provided. Transformative roles emerge from the spontaneous interaction of old and new to produce new meanings for old stories.

Chapter 6 completes this section by describing the types of dramas in the Therapeutic Spiral Model. Clinical contracts guide experiential methods to prevent uncontrolled regression and unconscious abreactions. In TSM, directing becomes a clinical job and the boundaries of the type of drama help to maintain conscious awareness as clients spiral into trauma bubbles to find new words to describe haunting images.

CHAPTER FOUR

The Action Trauma Team

CHAPTER OVERVIEW

This chapter presents the second clinical action structure of the Therapeutic Spiral Model, the action trauma team. It is my belief that the safest and deepest experiential group work with trauma survivors should not be done alone, if at all possible. It is too draining on the providers and not always contained enough for clients. This chapter describes the roles and functions of the members of a TSM action trauma team. It presents both the clinical and psychodramatic skills needed for competent practice in each role. Clients share how valuable their experience is with a team of trained professionals working together.

A primary clinical goal of all work in the Therapeutic Spiral Model is to prevent triggering uncontrolled regression and unconscious abreaction with experiential methods. The primitive defenses and vulnerable self-organization of most trauma survivors must be treated with respect when using action methods, in order to prevent the risk of retraumatization.

In the TSM this is done, most carefully, through the use of an action trauma team. This is a clinical team that is trained to use the modified psychodrama methods of TSM with trauma survivors. Each clinician is educated in traditional methods of healing (medicine, psychology, social work, counseling, education, expressive arts, advocacy, mediation, law, etc.). Usually they have received some additional graduate training in experiential psychotherapy, most often classical psychodrama or Gestalt therapy, before they start training in the Therapeutic Spiral Model.

An action trauma team in the Therapeutic Spiral Model includes trained clinicians in the roles of

- team leader (TL),
- assistant leader (AL), and
- trained auxiliary egos (TAE).

Together, the functions of these team roles work to co-create a safe container for clients. With support they can choose to slowly and consciously access unprocessed trauma bubbles with experiential methods. Dissociated emotions can be experienced and expressed. Life-affirming endings can be given to haunting memories. New narrative labels are formed in the present with the help of a trained clinical team.

During one workshop, Tricia asked to do a confrontation with her grandfather. Peter (TAE) played the perpetrator role for her. Ann (TAE) was her guardian angel. Mario (TL) directed the drama while Colette (AL) worked with the group to integrate everyone into the action as needed. It was a full team effort and Tricia stated, "I have never felt so safe before. I knew I could trust Peter to play that role and not hurt me and Ann was a godsend as my angel. I did have an angel back then. Today, I really got to feel her."

ROLES OF THE ACTION TRAUMA TEAMS

Each TSM team role incorporates clinical considerations within a psychodramatic framework. Team interventions work together to help clients spiral into unprocessed trauma bubbles for increased experiencing, and spiral back out into new words. The action trauma team strives to ensure safe experiential treatment with PTSD.

TEAM LEADER

The team leader's primary job in the TSM is to be the clinical director for the client that is the protagonist. Second to that, it is the director's responsibility to interface constantly with the assistant leader and trained auxiliary egos to use the interventions made possible by an action trauma team. In that way, the TSM promotes the deepest level of developmental repair possible for all group members.

A team leader can allow the chaos of the trauma survivor's inner world to be externalized in TSM by using containment or expansion intervention modules as clinically indicated. The team leader makes directing decisions based on clinical information about the level of adaptive functioning and goals of the session. In the TSM, clinical knowledge of diagnosis, treatment plans, transference, and psychological resiliency balance the timing, intensity, depth, and duration of all psychodramatic interventions.

Clinical Skills

There are three clinical skills that are crucial for the team leader working with trauma using experiential methods. They are the abilities to

1) conduct ongoing process assessment during a session,
2) use targeted intervention modules to contain unconscious regression and unconscious abreaction, and
3) promote narrative labeling at all times.

When these three clinical principles guide the use of action methods in the Therapeutic Spiral Model, safety is ensured.

Ongoing Process Assessment. The ability to track the moment by moment changes in clients is one of the most important clinical skills with experiential methods. As Greenberg (2001) notes, experiential therapy includes task-directed interventions. Interventions are implemented when the therapist assesses that the client is ready. In the Therapeutic Spiral Model, the three strands of the spiral begin the process of tracking clients in the here and now.

Diagnosis. Issues of diagnosis affect which intervention module to implement as well. When treating someone with a mood disorder symptom, such as depression with negative self-statements, a method that interrupts this pattern of thinking should be used. When working with someone diagnosed with borderline personality disorder, uncontrolled rage and negative transference can be expected as part of the healing process.

In the TSM, medical diagnosis does not create a psychopathology that becomes iatrogenic and self-reinforcing. Diagnosis is merely a useful tool for communicating how a certain set of trauma symptoms present in a client's life. In some cases, like with alcoholism and drug addiction, diagnosis may suggest some pre-therapy work, such as detoxification, a 12-step program, or inpatient treatment.

Andrea clearly suffered the symptoms of PTSD. The fact that she was also diagnosed with anorexia, a life threatening problem, however, informed the clinical process for using TSM with her. The team leader implemented interventions such as the body double (see chapter 5) to focus on positive body awareness so she could maintain a conscious state free of body memories and flashbacks. Whenever she worked, the body double would help contain her dissociation from her body and help her label what was happening. An example follows:

Andrea: I hate my body. It is disgusting and I never want to eat again!

Team Leader: Let me help you with these feelings by putting in a body double as extra support for you, OK? The body double talks like part of you—in the first person. The body double helps you remember when you did feel OK about your body. Can you pick someone to take this role? (She picks Ann [TAE] for the role. She steps in and immediately begins to produce information for Mario to work with as team leader).

Body Double: Even when I feel like this, I can notice my breath, the breath of life. It's not really my body that is the problem, it is what happened to my body that hurts.

Andrea: Yes, yes I know it is about what happened, the rape. I used to love my body. Now I hate it.

Team Leader: Listen to your body double and if she is right repeat the words, even if the experience seems like long ago.

Body Double: I do feel like I hate my body now, but I also remember when I loved it . . . before the rape. Maybe now I can just take one deep breath and feel the aliveness of my life force today.

Process Diagnosis.   The second type of assessment skills that are crucial for the team leader are process skills. You must be able to assess, in the moment, how the protagonist and group members' adaptive capacities are holding up and to adjust your clinical decisions accordingly. Is there too much energy? If so, then use interventions that contain and decrease intrusive affects and memories. Are there enough positive roles to support increased experiencing? If yes, then ask the protagonist to concretize a trauma scene in the circle of scarves. Is the person getting overwhelmed with feelings? Suggest a meaning making intervention. The three strands of the spiral provide a basis for process assessment and help to guide clinical decision making throughout TSM dramas.

When Vladamir was confronting the auxiliaries playing the soldiers who kidnapped his family, he was emotionally triggered into out-of-control rage. He had been fine one moment; the next moment he was pacing, shouting, and loudly hitting one fist with another. The team leader told him to "hold" and gave him a containing double as support (see chapter 5). Then he could address the perpetrators without losing control of his affect and energy.

Containing Regression and Abreaction. When the team leader assesses the prescriptive roles to be in place, the client is ready to work directly with information in trauma bubbles. The use of an action trauma team, guided by the team leader, is integral to the safety needed for controlled regression and conscious expression of affect. Regression is used in TSM work with trauma survivors, but only in the service of the ego. That means that the team leader must structure all regressive work so that it does not overwhelm the defenses and adaptive capacity of protagonist and/or group members. If the protagonist *chooses* to consciously reexperience a younger ego state or to express dissociated feelings, only then does the team leader facilitate emotional expression.

When Jim began to feel like a little boy when he was watching someone else's drama, the team leader asked the assistant leader to work with him on the sidelines to help him stay in his adult state. Later, in his own drama, Mario directed him to role reverse into his 8-year-old self:

TL: Jim, can you please pick someone to be little Jimmy. [He chooses Peter, a TAE.] Now role reverse and become your 8-year-old self, talking to your adult self.

Jim as 8-year-old self: I am really hurting. I feel like I just can't grow up. I'm stuck here in the past with Dad. Can you help me?

TL: Reverse roles and speak back from your adult role.

Jim as adult self: I can help. That's why I'm here today doing this work—so you can get better and grow up and stop running my life. I'm the adult. I'll take care of you now. I am in the process of creating a safe life and world for you.

Promoting Narrative Labeling. The third important clinical skill for the team leader to have is to be able to promote narrative labeling at all times with experiential methods. All too often in classical psychodrama, the director goes directly for affect regardless of whether the protagonist is maintaining cognitive capacity or not. With the TSM, the team leader works to maintain a balance between affective experiencing and meaning making at all times, in order to not retraumatize clients.

When Andrea was completing a TSM drama, talking directly to the boys who had raped her, the TL role reversed her back and forth from her observing ego card on the wall to the child role that carried all the unprocessed rage. When she began to get triggered emotionally, he would immediately put her in the observing role. When she got too cognitive there and lost touch with her feelings, she was reversed back to the child role. These interventions by the team leader were crucial to keeping her anchored in the present and fully conscious of what she was saying and doing.

Psychodrama Skills

The TSM team leader must also be an expert in using experiential methods. Clinicians are trained in classical psychodrama, Gestalt therapy, and the modified intervention modules of the Therapeutic Spiral Model. Three psychodrama skills that are crucial to the safe enactment of trauma scenes are the ability to:

- direct a psychodrama,
- direct a team, and
- structure safe affective expression.

When these three psychodrama skills are combined with clinical knowledge, TSM dramas can provide for developmental repair of even the most horrendous stories of trauma and abuse.

Directing a Psychodrama. The classical psychodrama structure of warm-up, action, and sharing is translated into the three strands of the spiral image for consistency and ease of use.

Energy—The Warm-Up. The warm-up builds energy and safety as described in chapter 3. The team leader decides which action interventions to use for assessment, connection, and narrative labeling prior to beginning any direct trauma work. The team leader also directs the process of choosing a protagonist.

In classical psychodrama there are many ways to select which person will tell a story of trauma at a certain time in a group (see Blatner, 2000). In the Therapeutic Spiral Model, we most often choose a protagonist based on self-selection and group support and readiness. What that means is that the team leader asks, "Who wants to put their story into action today?"

Group members who are willing to be the protagonist step into the circle of scarves. Each person shares a bit of his or her story and the team leader paraphrases it in terms of a clinical goal. For instance,

Andrea: I'd like to work on being in my body today. I have been able to stop some of my self-hatred, so I guess I'd like to see what it feels like to stop cutting off my body from my mind and my heart.

Team Leader: OK, your work would be about finding some positive feelings in your body today? Having a good experience as you come back into your body?

Jim: What I want is to confront my father for all his years of abuse. I am finally mad at him rather than mad at myself, and I really want to get all this rage I've been carrying out of my system tonight.

Team Leader: So, you would be contracting to do a scene where you would release your rage, the rage that has been dissociated all these years? You would do that safely and with support.

Tricia: I'd like to figure out what these body memories are trying to tell me. I mean, I was fine for 35 years and now all of a sudden I have flashbacks and body memories at the merest trigger.

Team Leader: You want to find some words to connect your body and your mind? You want to understand and have new narrative labels about what is happening to you now and how it connects to the past?

At this point, the team leader asks the group members to choose the story that will help them the most if they see it enacted that day. They use action sociograms to make the choices in action, putting their hand on the shoulder of the person whose issue will help them the most. The person with the most hands is the protagonist, if that person is making a choice for self-support. That way, the protagonist is willing to work and the group support is there to make it safe.

Each individual psychodrama also has a warm-up scene, that in the TSM, is always a scene where the prescriptive roles are enacted to increase strengths and containment. After a clinical contract for the type of drama, the team leader uses the warm-up scene to increase the energy of roles of restoration, containment, and observation prior to enacting trauma-based scenes.

Experiencing—Action. Action is the part of the psychodrama that focuses on increased experiencing and affective expression. The team leader uses the multitude of psychodramatic methods and interventions available to enact one or more scenes to explore trauma and create developmental repair.

As the majority of the rest of this book details the action of a TSM drama, suffice it to say at this point, that one of the team leader's main responsibilities is to follow the trauma survivor's intrapsychic role atom (see chapter 5) to enact trauma-based scenes safely. Scene 1 always develops prescriptive roles. After they are stabilized, the team leader may enact a number of trauma-based scenes. In this way, regression is controlled and in the service of the ego.

Surplus reality scenes complete the action part of most TSM dramas. Together with the protagonist, the team leader creates a scene of developmental repair. In one drama, Andrea got to stage a scene of justice and restitution where she picked people to play the judge and jury who sentenced the boys who gang-raped her to life in prison. She did not want the death penalty because she "had more respect for life than that."

In another drama, Vladamir talks to his mother in a wished for conversation. He tells her he is sorry and is able to experience her forgiveness through the auxiliary playing the role. This scene frees his heart from the relentless guilt that been pounding him for a year.

Sharing—Meaning Making.   The team leader directs sharing, the final part of any psychodrama. Each person shares the insights they gained from the roles they played in the protagonist's drama. Sharing provides the opportunity for narrative labeling and meaning making for all. People have a chance to connect how a role they played is relevant to their lives. The protagonist has a chance to sit back and feel connected to the group. Shared experience becomes shared meaning to carry into the future.

Directing a Team.   A second important psychodrama skill is the ability to direct a team of auxiliaries with an assistant leader. While the AL role is unique to the Therapeutic Spiral Model, working with auxiliaries is a long tradition in classical psychodrama. In most cases group members benefit greatly from playing roles in other people's dramas, but having a group of clinically trained role players is a rich resource of creativity and surplus reality.

The Therapeutic Spiral Model is always conducted with a team even if it is only a team of two people. Thus, the team leader must be able to not only direct a protagonist in enacting his or her story, the TL must also be able to direct a team to work together in the best possible manner. There are many fine nuances of this team director role, with the guiding statement of responsibility being that the TL interfaces with the assistant leader and trained auxiliary egos to support containment and controlled regression in the services of clients.

Together with the AL, the TL makes clinical decisions about the directing of the type of TSM drama that is contracted for. The TL directs the protagonist and the AL directs the group. Both have access to the TAEs for roles of support and containment.

Safe Expression of Affect. When working with trauma, the use of adaptive affects in the service of the ego is crucial. Clients must not be overwhelmed by intense emotions as they break out of trauma bubbles. They must be able to experience and express long dissociated feelings and memories in a safe and contained structure. Presented here are three classical psychodrama techniques that are regularly used by a team leader to create safe structures for intense emotion.

Bataca Work. Plastic bats covered with "nerf" material or other padding can be used as a prop when expressing anger and rage. The team leader sets up the scene and instructs the protagonist how to hold the bataca and how to use it safely—feet planted securely, bringing it up over one's head, and down on the cushion/chair/block.

The protagonist then hits a chair or pillow, with support from an auxiliary to remain fully conscious of what s/he is saying and expressing. Jim found his voice when he was doing bataca work in a drama, shouting at his father, "I told you it was you and not me. You did it. I was just an innocent kid. So now you can hear my anger!"

The Rage Hold. In TSM, team leaders teach the group how to use a rage hold ahead of time so that it can be a chosen intervention during the height of affective expression. This is a method of physical containment that provides a holding environment even for the most intense rage. It must be conducted only by trained practitioners.

Andrea was able to finally express the intense rage and hatred she felt at her perpetrators by using a rage hold. With the help of the team, she was contained and allowed to have an "adult temper tantrum" until she had exhausted herself. Then she turned to an auxiliary ego and told him, "I am done now. God, does my body feel different."

The Nurturing Hold.   This is a method of providing comfort and nurturing when people are experiencing intense grief or despair. An auxiliary ego holds the protagonist so that s/he is well supported physically and there is no uncomfortable touching. The team leader directs the protagonist to "lean into this support and have your feelings."

Tricia was able to let Ann (TAE) hold her one day and she sobbed for 15 minutes about how the flashbacks had interrupted her work as an attorney and really frightened her. She sounded like a motherless child and was gently soothed and comforted until her grief naturally abated.

The Therapeutic Spiral Model has a set of principles of conscious reexperiencing that structure the expression of intense affect even more fully. The TL directs the protagonist through a series of steps that promote controlled regression and conscious expression in a balanced experience of healing (see chapters 7–10).

ASSISTANT LEADER

It is a team effort to allow the protagonist to enact the chaos of the inner symbolic world. When the integration of group members who may become triggered is added to the mix, it is a full clinical job to do either/or for the team leader. Thus, the assistant leader role was created in the Therapeutic Spiral Model to provide additional support for the team leader and group members.

The assistant leader is the gatekeeper between the action of the director with the protagonist and any triggered trauma reactions among group members. As such, the AL is in continual motion, walking the perimeter of the circle of experiencing. S/he stays in an observing role and from this vantage point monitors and enhances the drama for safety.

While the director is constantly monitoring the safety of the protagonist in the progression of the drama, the assistant leader is concerned primarily with the safe implementation of all auxiliary roles among team and group members. Basically, the AL directs the team auxiliaries as the director works with the protagonist. Like the director, the assistant leader is both clinician and psychodramatist.

Clinical Skills

The risk of the protagonist's enactment triggering another group member is high when working experientially with a group of trauma survivors.

Having an AL allows all group members free expression of their responses without having to hide their experience from others.

Two clinical skills that are particular to the role of assistant leader in TSM are listed below:

1) supporting and integrating group members that are triggered by a protagonist's story, and
2) identification and enactment of projective identifications that are an assumption of this model of group psychotherapy.

Interventions With Group Members. The assistant leader assesses group members' levels of personal safety, positive roles, and interpersonal support throughout the drama. If a group member becomes triggered into primitive defenses such as dissociation, the AL can assign a TAE as a body double to interrupt the pattern. If a trauma bubble bursts, the AL can ask a TAE to be a containing double to balance cognition and emotion. The AL can also cluster group members that are having similar responses to a protagonist's story for support and containment.

When Jim went through a drama on confronting his father, a lot of group members were scared by his rage, even though they trusted him completely. The AL clustered people into three smaller groups: dissociation, terror, and defense of the perpetrator. This allowed all group members to have their responses without shame or blame.

Another clinical responsibility of the AL is to assess when to bridge the distance between the group member who is triggered by a protagonist's drama, and when to support the group member separately through trained auxiliaries. This can be done in an overt consultation with the TL. More often, the AL assesses the adaptive capacity of the group member and the timing in the drama. Then, s/he will "throw in" a spontaneous role as clinically indicated.

Tricia participated in six experiential weekends as part of her TSM treatment plan. During her first workshop, she sat fairly stoically throughout most of the dramas, no matter how intensely she was experiencing things. However, one could see she was depleted, lonely, and emotionally hurting.

In her second "Surviving Spirits" workshop, the assistant leader put Tricia in a cluster of people that were trying to take care of others, rather than focusing on themselves. She coached the group to make statements communicating, "I have needs. My needs are important. I can ask for what I want." During the sharing, Tricia cried as she spoke quietly about how her needs were never taken seriously when she was growing up. She told of how she had learned from her mother to take care of everyone else's needs first. Today, she knows that her needs are equally important.

Enacting Projective Identifications.   Trauma bubbles do burst. A group member spontaneously erupts into feelings, or dissociates, or acts out uncontrollably. This unprocessed information automatically and unconsciously becomes projected during group work with trauma survivors. Chaos can result.

In TSM, feelings and actions are integrated into the action through the healthy, clinical use of projective identifications (PI). The assistant leader identifies the PI and encourages a team member to take the role on so it can be concretized in the protagonist's space. When clinically guided by the AL, this action sequence prevents group members from collapsing in shame spirals or bursting out in rage.

Enacting PIs can result in a vast integration of clinical information from trauma bubbles that were dissociated, disembodied, and defended against during the conscious reexperiencing of trauma material. Working in tandem with the AL and TAE, the team leader can help the protagonist to claim or reject these dissociated experiences through many action interventions.

Andrea learned to work well with the process of projective identification in her group. She contracted to do a conscious reexperiencing drama around the rage she still felt. The entire group felt the intensity of her PIs that were floating around the room. Even though Andrea could label her experience as rage, her psychological awareness could only hold so much affect, and the group members picked up on what was left, according to their own identification.

As the team leader helped Andrea set up on the stage the roles of the boys who had gang-raped her using the TAEs, the AL organized the group members into supportive roles of anger expression. As Andrea expressed her rage in a rage hold, other group members beat on drums. A few hit the chair with batacas.

Still others pounded their feet as they raised their voices in cleansing sounds of righteous indignation. Finally, a symphony of power came out of the cacophony. The assistant leader directed the sub-scenes while the team leader directed the protagonist, as the group spiraled out of primary process and into new shared meaning. The final outcome was one of beauty as the protagonist and group declared, "I have my power back."

Psychodrama Skills

In a TSM drama, it is the assistant leader role that ultimately determines whether the chaos becomes overwhelming to individuals and the group or is channeled into the healing energy of the therapeutic spiral. With the use of trained auxiliary egos, the assistant leader works to provide safety at the deepest levels of psychodramatic experiencing for all group members.

Shared Directing.   The AL codirects the trained auxiliary egos to implement the director's interventions through use of the team. S/he integrates spontaneous auxiliary roles from group members and team members. S/he makes therapeutic role assignments for people in the audience.

While the assistant leader assesses safety and makes group interventions as needed, the team leader can continue to direct the protagonist's drama without interruption. The AL directs the team members that are not actively in roles for the protagonist, and thus can provide support for clients that are being triggered.

Directing Sub-Scenes.   The AL may also direct a side scene that is integrated into the action of the protagonist at a later moment in the drama. An important psychodramatic skill for the assistant leader is knowing when to have a triggered group member enter the action of the drama, and when to work with this person on the side (Burger, personal communication, October 28, 2001). Timing of sub-scenes is crucial to maintaining the balance between cognition and affect, and not overwhelming the group with too much chaos.

Once when Jim was triggered by someone else's drama, the AL chose to work with him on the sidelines to ground and center him. In another workshop, he was triggered into rage as he watched a protagonist cower in front of her father who had abused her. In this case, the AL assessed that Jim's rage was a PI and was appropriate to the action. The AL directed Jim to take his anger up on the stage and offer it to the protagonist to counteract the depletion of terror. Then, the TL could role reverse them both for a new experience to break trauma patterns.

TRAINED AUXILIARY EGOS

Trained auxiliary egos (TAEs) are a rich resource for the action trauma team, the protagonist, and the group. They provide safety when working with unprocessed information, especially when the contract is for conscious reexperiencing of past core trauma scenes.

In classical psychodrama the auxiliary ego serves three primary functions and two deeper functions (Moreno, Z. T., 1965). These are:

1) to take on the role required by the protagonist,
2) to represent the protagonist's perception of the role, and
3) to explore the protagonist's material in action.

The deeper functions are 4) to give additional information about which the protagonist may not be consciously aware, and 5) to offer guidance and instruction. It is within these last two role functions, and beyond, that auxiliaries trained in the Therapeutic Spiral Model function most fully.

The main job of TAEs is to facilitate the process of the protagonist's enactment and group members' level of experiencing as directed by both the team leader and the assistant leader. There are three main psychological functions trained auxiliary egos serve in the therapeutic spiral model:

1) TAEs provide containment to group members who are triggered.
2) TAEs utilize projective identifications by putting them into an active role in the drama.
3) TAEs play difficult or potentially re-traumatizing roles such as victim or perpetrator as needed.

If the AL is the gatekeeper of information, then the TAEs are the runners that provide assessments of safety at any moment in a drama.

Clinical Skills

Three clinical skills that TAEs need to be well trained with, in using experiential methods with trauma survivors, are the abilities to:

1) provide clinical methods of containment,
2) identify and enact projective identifications, and
3) structure controlled regression in the service of the ego.

Creating Containment.　A primary clinical function of a trained auxiliary is to work with the team leader and AL to implement experiential interventions at clinical choice points for containment with trauma survivors. When the protagonist's story triggers flashbacks, uncontrolled abreaction, primitive defenses or ego state shifts in other group members, TAEs are invaluable to the safety of the group and the uninterrupted production of the drama. A TAE can work separately and quietly with a triggered group member to orient and anchor that person into the present reality through a body or containing double or other intervention modules.

When Jim went to his first Surviving Spirits workshop, he became triggered the first night, when the participants were naming their traumas. The AL noticed this starting to happen, and directed a TAE to go stand beside Jim and help him focus on the here and now, rather than the there and then. He was assigned a containing double, a prescriptive role in TSM.

The action continued with people stepping in to admit that they had been sexually abused, physically abused, emotionally abandoned; that they had alcoholic fathers; that they had mothers who were manic-depressive or schizophrenic. Jim could participate and attend to the task of narrative labeling with auxiliary support.

Containment interventions are used quite often in the Therapeutic Spiral Model to maintain the safety of experiential methods with trauma survivors. During a TSM drama, TAEs are often used as support for group members playing other roles so they can maintain full conscious awareness of all that they say and do.

This happened when Colette (TAE) spontaneously enacted the prescriptive role of the manager of defenses in a drama with Vladamir. Rather than letting the group get caught in a sense of dissociation, the TAE therapeutically used it to change the energy of this defense into positive containment. She created a bag from extra scarves. This container was to hold dissociation. She went around and engaged with each person she saw beginning to leave the here and now, and had them put their dissociation into the bag.

Enacting Projective Identifications. When the AL decides to expand the action through the use of TAEs, they are most often clinically intervening to enact projective identifications. When enacted, PIs can be integrated into the drama rather than floating around and triggering other group members. TAEs learn how to identify PIs and put them into action as needed, to help control the chaos of primary process enactments of trauma bubbles.

The clinical skills involved in being able to identify PIs and decide how to use them to increase the protagonist's awareness has many components (see chapter 11). TAEs take unconscious information that is projected and dissociated into the room and concretize it through action and nonverbal behavior. Then the group can benefit from this process rather than it resulting in chaos.

When Vladamir enacted a drama confronting the Bosnian soldiers about the rape and murder of his mothers and sisters, one could feel a tight tension in the room. Two psychologists from Bosnia were also part of the multicultural training group. Two of the TAEs on the team picked up on the PIs floating around the room and spontaneously staged a moment's scene to modulate and name the affect:

TAE1:   I am hatred. I am fear. I am the evil lord of dark emotions. I belong to all of you. Become my prey. Hate, rape, murder . . . be like me. I hate everyone. I want to destroy life.

TAE2 in response: And I am a warrior of truth. I am a lighted being that sees the fear that causes humans to hurt each other. You may cause the fear, but I can show them courage.

In this enactment, the unspoken fears and the generational hatred and anxieties were all given voice. The metaphorical use of mythic figures goes beyond the individuals in the room, or even the nationalities and their history. The situation became, in that moment, a universal theme of good and evil.

The team leader had many options at that point on how to proceed. This is where the finesse of the clinically trained auxiliary ego in the Therapeutic Spiral Model comes into play. Action structures are used as clinical interventions in trauma-based patterns for individuals and groups.

Regression in the Service of the Ego.   TAEs provide the clinical support for controlled regression into victim, perpetrator, and abandoning authority roles (see chapter 9). In order to do so, TAEs learn to identify their own countertransference, trauma triggers, and interpersonal difficulties. They learn to use their own trauma material in the service of the client from any role that they are given.

Victim Role.   Unless there is a clinical reason for further exploration of the victim role (such as memory retrieval, state dependent learning, affect expression, or role transformation), trained auxiliary egos enact the victim role in all conscious reexperiencing scenes and child role interactions.

On the other hand, when the victim role is resourced, the client can begin to experience this state though the image of the wounded child. The wounded child role gives a name to the state that holds the experience of the original trauma when development was frozen. This name decreases some of the shame many survivors feel as a result of horror and helplessness at the time of trauma. With support, even the most painful victim experiences can be repaired.

One of Jim's most intense psychodramas focused on consciously reexperiencing memories of being violently physically abused at age 5 by his father in an alcoholic rage, and then running to a favorite uncle for help, only to be brutally sodomized by him. While he could intellectually understand how that particular abuse could result in intense rage, he could not truly accept that this was "righteous" rage. When he witnessed his child self in terror, he was able to make integrated meaning of his experience.

This scene was safely experienced by having Peter, a TAE play the wounded child role of 5-year-old Jim. Mark, an AE in training, played the uncle. As Jim watched his 5-year-old child run to his uncle, only to start to be sexually assaulted, he stood up and screamed "Stop." This new action interrupted the original scene and created a new reparative ending.

Perpetrator Roles. At some point in the Therapeutic Spiral Model, it may be clinically indicated for a client to play perpetrator roles in order to reclaim personal power, disrupt identification with the aggressor, or discriminate one's own abusive behaviors. When the protagonist has the ego strength and spontaneity to actively experience the role of perpetrator, valuable unconscious information can be unlocked.

When clients can move in and out of the roles of perpetrators, there is a sense of mastery and reclaiming of personal power that may have been given to the perpetrator for survival. Playing a perpetrator role is structured in TSM (see chapter 10) with a TAE initially taking the role and then supporting the protagonist to do so. This is a crucial difference from classical psychodrama. In TSM, people do not take the perpetrator role until clinically indicated. Tricia asked Ann (TAE) to play the role of her alcoholic mother when it was too overwhelming to play it herself. In this session, the TAE as drunken mother stumbled around the room, and played this perpetrator role with just the right element of command and comedy. Tricia was able to see the many ways her mother's alcoholism had impacted her. When the role had lost some of its power through the TAE portrayal, Tricia was then able to fully reverse roles and show mastery over this internalized perpetrator role. TAEs are built into the safe enactment of both victim and perpetrator roles, and help promote healing at the deepest levels of psychodramatic work in the Therapeutic Spiral Model.

Psychodrama Skills

TAEs are also trained at basic psychodrama skills when they are accredited at this level in the Therapeutic Spiral Model. They know the basic psychodrama techniques and when to use them. Additionally, they are trained in the prescriptive roles of TSM as action structures, not just as clinical tools. Many TAEs have a background in the performing arts or creative pursuits, at varied levels of professional training.

Action Demands.   Auxiliaries know how to put action demands on the protagonist from a dramatic perspective. From a role, the TAE pulls for a certain reciprocal role to test out a clinical hypothesis or interrupt a trauma-based pattern. This is called putting an action demand on the protagonist, because one is demanding a certain return action to the role taken, i.e., mother and child, victim and perpetrator.

At one moment in Vladamir's drama, his rage edged close to being out of control. Peter (TAE) was in role as a soldier and noticed this concern as a clinician. In that moment, he turned to his "troops" and said, "Calm down a minute men . . . this guy looks like he's gonna blow." In this way, the TAE took an action from a role that demanded some new response from both his fellow teammates (the other soldiers) and from the protagonist. He alerted his team members to a potentially explosive emotion and he helped Vladamir to take a moment and put cognitive labels on what he was experiencing.

Playing Difficult Roles.   A significant psychodrama function of a trained auxiliary ego is to play roles that the protagonist or group members experience as too difficult, emotionally overwhelming, or ego threatening. The two main role clusters that many trauma survivors find difficult to enact are the victim and perpetrator roles. TAEs enact these difficult roles until clients learn how to experience unconscious trauma material as stated above. They draw on training in improvisation, spontaneity, drama, and other expressive arts to make the roles true to life and yet not overwhelming to clients.

FUNCTIONS OF THE ACTION TRAUMA TEAM

This chapter has separated each of the roles of the action trauma team into component clinical and psychodramatic skills. The team leader, the assistant leader, and the trained auxiliaries work together and at many times their skills overlap. To complete this team description I want to end by looking at the four functions of a director in classical psychodrama. In TSM, the team is ultimately the director and all roles share director's functions.

Kellermann (1992) described the psychodrama director's role as composed of four distinct, yet integrated, functions: analyst, therapist, group leader, and producer. All team members learn and practice these clinical functions and enact them in their designated team roles as part of all TSM dramas.

ANALYST

The clinical function of the analyst role is to analyze any therapeutic situation, to break it into parts and weigh the variables, and to provide a certain outcome. It is this analytic function of the therapist that ensures clinical safety in the TSM.

THERAPIST

All team members must be practitioners who are clinically astute, psychologically flexible, and sincerely sensitive at the interpersonal level. This is especially so with trauma survivors whose defenses for self-preservation may be overdeveloped, making trust and building a therapeutic alliance slow going in the beginning of therapy.

Transference difficulties also trigger uncontrolled regression as part of any therapeutic relationship, but can be more intense with experiential methods, if not contained in the therapeutic alliance. The task-directive stance of the experiential therapist can only be used with full informed consent inside a well-developed therapeutic relationship.

GROUP LEADER/SOCIOMETRIST

As sociometrist, the team helps build group cohesion and trust which are necessary to maintain a group or workshop. Often, shame, fear, and distrust have kept many clients with PTSD isolated for years, and the need to build trusting relationships is primary. It is truly a special moment of healing when a protagonist sits back and relaxes in sharing and says, "Oh, I'm *not* alone!"

Another important sociometric function specific to the TSM is how to include all group participants in the action of the drama. Group members are encouraged, and it eventually becomes a group norm, to trust their spontaneity and let themselves actively experience their self-organization in the present moment. For some clients that will mean pacing the floor in rage. For others it is to externalize the struggle to stay present or to dissociate to the ceiling. At all times, the team works together to find ways to promote inclusion of these feelings. The team lives the motto "no shame no blame."

PRODUCER

The producer is the most clearly dramatic function of the action trauma team in the Therapeutic Spiral Model. It is in the production, in the staging of the scenes, in the action that happens that the spontaneity of the team leader and team becomes most visible. The function of producer is seen most clearly in this model through the clinical action structures developed for affective management and conscious reexperiencing to promote developmental repair. Team members constantly assess the physical and psychological safety of the group and produce clinical action structures to support either containment or expression. Boundaries can be concretized with scarves, feelings can be structured for expression, and interpersonal connections made for support.

CONCLUSIONS

When the action trauma team functions as a well-put-together entity, it becomes the archetypal, collective "psychodramatic director." With this concept, the individual director of a particular drama does not have sole responsibility for all the director's functions. In the TSM, the drama enacted and the healing which ensues become the shared responsibility of the action trauma team as a whole (Toscani, 1993). Participants, in both clinical and training groups, who have experienced the sound working of the action trauma team have unequivocally commented on the power and safety of its use.

CHAPTER FIVE

The Trauma Survivor's Intrapsychic Role Atom: A Clinical Map For Action

CHAPTER OVERVIEW

This chapter presents the third clinical action structure of the Therapeutic Spiral Model. It is called the trauma survivor's intrapsychic role atom (TSIRA) and was developed in collaboration with several of my colleagues (Cossa & Hudgins, 1998; Hudgins, 2000; Toscani & Hudgins, 1996). The Three-Child Model of Recovery (Sheridan & Hudgins, 1990) is the earlier template of the present intrapsychic role atom.

The TSIRA provides a clinical map for the enactment of all roles in TSM. It guides the sequence and enactment of all action intervention modules to prevent uncontrolled regression. Prescriptive roles for observation, restoration, and containment are always enacted in a TSM drama. Only then can trauma-based roles be consciously reexperienced. Out of this spontaneous interaction emerges the roles of personal transformation.

DESCRIPTION OF THE TRAUMA SURVIVOR'S INTRAPSYCHIC ROLE ATOM

In classical psychodrama there are a number of assessment tools to measure interpersonal relationships. The social atom shows the minimum number of relationships needed for someone to maintain homeostasis (Moreno, 1977). The cultural atom examines the roles that are internalized and then enacted in reciprocal interpersonal relationships (Clayton, L., 1982; McVea, 1997).

In TSM, the trauma survivor's intrapsychic role atom (TSIRA) is a clinical map of the essential internal roles in the self-organization and personality structure of a trauma survivor. It shows the impact of trauma on self-organization as defined by role theory. The TSIRA is divided into three categories of roles:

1) prescriptive roles—those roles that are needed in place for healthy personality functioning,
2) trauma-based roles—those roles that were internalized from traumatic experiences, and
3) transformative roles—those roles that develop from the spontaneous interaction of trauma-based and prescriptive roles.

When these roles are followed in the clinical order indicated in TSM, experiential methods can be used safely and easily. Role terms make the TSIRA user friendly to clients, while therapists find a clinical map useful for containment.

PRESCRIPTIVE ROLES

Working with the prescriptive roles for PTSD is pre-trauma work. Prescriptive roles serve three main psychological functions for the protagonist, group, family, or organization:

1) observation,
2) restoration, and
3) containment.

When the prescriptive roles are developed, clients have reached the TSM defined state of spontaneous learning and are able to directly work with unprocessed trauma material.

Roles of Observation

The first set of prescriptive roles that are concretized in TSM address the ability to be able to neutrally observe self without shame or blame. Only when behaviors can be seen clearly can they be changed. There are two observing roles that are clinical in nature, and can be assigned by the team leader as needed: a) the observing ego, and b) the client role.

Purpose: To build and sustain an integrated state of spontaneous learning.
Cossa and Hudgins (1998) have created this table to summarize the TSIRA (Toscani & Hudgins, 1996). Yorke (personal communication, Sept. 16, 1997) introduced the term "spontaneous learning state."

PRESCRIPTIVE ROLES

Strengths

Function: **Restoration**	Function: **Containment**	Function: **Observation**
Personal	Body Double	Observing Ego
Interpersonal	Containing Double	Client Role
Transpersonal	Keeper of the Defenses	

⇨ An Integrated State of Spontaneity

⇨ Change-Agent Role

TRAUMA-BASED ROLES

Holder of Defenses

Defenses

Function: **Survival**	Function: **Compensation**	Function: **Communication**
Dissociation	Maladaptive Roles	Victim Roles
Denial	Obsessions	Perpetrator Roles
Multiple States of Consciousness	Compulsions	Abandoning Authority
Idealization	Addictions	
Projective Identification		
Identification With Aggressor		

PRESCRIPTIVE ROLES AND TRAUMA-BASED ROLES ⇨ Conscious Reexperiencing with Narrative Labeling

⇨ Manager of Healthy Functioning

TRANSFORMATIVE ROLES

Function: **Autonomy**	Function: **Connection**	Function: **Integration**
Sleeping-Awakening Child	Good-Enough Parent	Good-Enough Spirituality
Change Agent	Good-Enough Significant Other	
Manager of Healthy Functioning		

TRANSFORMATIVE ROLES ⇨ DEVELOPMENTAL REPAIR

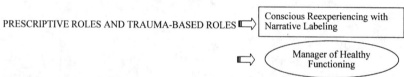

FIGURE 5.1 The trauma survivor's intrapsychic role atom summary (Cossa & Hudgins, 1998).

The Observing Ego (OE). This role represents a part of the ego that is able to neutrally observe thoughts, feelings, and actions. The observing ego is a clinical term for a role that remains emotionally neutral to what is happening and can simply "collect the facts" and "see the data without judgement."

As noted in chapter 3, OE cards are the first intervention in a Surviving Spirits workshop. Cards with symbols for power, angels, children, animals, and flowers, etc., are used each day in the workshop, so that the OE role continues to grow and develop. This intervention also marks a physical space for the OE role so it is available for role reversal if needed.

When Tricia was doing a regressive scene from the role of her wounded child, she began to unconsciously reexperience the terror she felt with her godfather who abused her. She quickly froze and started to shake. The TL role reversed her into her OE, represented by an angel card on the wall. She said,

OE/angel card: I am here to witness you today. You are not alone. I am holding an angel card and it says to focus on your intent to find your light. Your intent today is to stop the darkness . . . to stop the flashbacks from Sidney's physical and sexual abuse of you. I won't let you stay in that place anymore. Take my hand.

In wounded child role: I'm scared. He looks so big.

OE: But I am big now too. Look at me and take my hand.

Wounded child: OK, I can see you. You are an adult. I can see you have power. OK, I'll come over and stand beside you and take your hand.

Client Role. The client role was created as separate from the protagonist role specifically to work with people in a dissociated state. This role holds the function of the executive ego in TSM. It remains stable and focuses on the whole scene, while the protagonist role reverses into as many roles as needed. This role can be prescribed whenever regressive work is to be done to maintain object constancy.

When Jim contracted to do a conscious reexperiencing drama, the TL asked him to pick someone to be his "client self—the part of you that came here to do the work, no matter how hard it gets." This role was then available to him when he chose to reexperience his own 5-year-old self, later in the drama. The auxiliary in the role kept saying, "It's OK. I can see everything that is happening and you are safe today."

Roles of Restoration

Restorative roles focus on enlivening the depleted trauma-based self, so that change can occur. This second cluster of prescriptive roles helps clients to feel more resilient, connected to others, and connected to a sense that there is something greater than self. For some people restoration may need to start with inpatient treatment, addiction recovery, medical intervention, or social welfare. After these basic needs are addressed, the psychological task is to actively experience internal roles of autonomy, self-support, and healthy connection to others in preparation for direct trauma work. For trauma survivors to be fully spontaneous and self-supported, restorative roles must be available at three levels of strengths:

1) personal,
2) interpersonal, and
3) transpersonal.

Personal Strengths. These roles can be any personal strengths that the clients can identify. When naming these strengths, the TL has the protagonist put them into a role for increased awareness and experiencing, for instance a courageous lion, a determined warrior, a brilliant teacher. When clients role reverse with these strengths they increase their state of spontaneity and feel empowered.

Even when clients say they have no strengths, the TL can ask them to mark a spot or an empty chair for a strength they would like to develop. They can still give it a role description and practice the role even if they don't believe it is a strength currently. Vladamir asked another group member to be his "competent psychologist" role when the TL asked the group to pick personal strengths for their art project. Andrea picked someone to be her "beautiful body." Tricia said she wanted her "aggressive litigator," and Jim picked a "serene peacemaker" for his personal strength.

Interpersonal Strengths. Even though TSM focuses on intrapsychic processes, protagonists need to have an internalized "other" to walk with them in a TSM drama. This role can be a real or imagined other, alive or dead, for example a good mother, a loving grandmother, a supportive spouse, a loyal dog, a shining hero from a book, a famous celebrity such as Oprah Winfrey. Abstract strengths that assist in interpersonal relationships, such as honesty, trust, and communication can also be enacted. As with personal strengths, it is necessary to develop a role for the strength to be translated for enactment, like an honest spouse, a trusting puppy, or a communication officer.

As Andrea set up her prescriptive roles in preparation to confront the boys who raped her, she asked Peter (TAE) to play her father, who she described as kind, loving, and "always on my side." This was their dialogue as the role was stabilized in the first scene:

Andrea: Dad, I feel like a little girl and I need you to be here with me. I don't think I can go back and confront those boys without your help.

Dad: Honey, you know I am always here for you. I am on your side at all times. In fact, let me stand beside you right now so you can feel me here. Is it OK if I put my arm around your shoulders?

Andrea: Yes, please. It is good to feel you physically present. Sometimes when I'm alone I imagine you are here with me. It feels good today to physically have you here as my auxillary.

Dad: Yes, I will walk by your side today. Together you and I will confront these boys and I will protect you. I am sorry I was not there when it happened to stop them then, but we will stop them today.

Transpersonal Strengths.   When trauma happens, human abilities cannot prevent it. The third restorative role is thus a transpersonal strength. This is a crucial element in TSM—to create a role for spirituality. When this happens, clients gain a sense of restoration that makes meaning of trauma in new ways. It can be nature, God, a higher power, music—something that is beyond what is human.

Like many people in 12-step programs, Jim could immediately embrace his transpersonal strength by concretizing his higher power. He asked Vladamir to play "HP" in one drama and used shiny gold and teal scarves to dress him in "colors of light and healing." As HP, Vladamir said, "You can always depend on me. I can change what you cannot. Seek me through prayer and meditation. Even when you forget me, I am with you. I love you unconditionally."

Roles of Containment

The third set of prescriptive roles provides containment for trauma survivors using action methods. Containment is a psychological term to describe a sense of emotional "holding" to support clients to stay in the present moment with cognitive and emotional processes balanced. Containment provides flexible yet solid boundaries.

Containing roles attempt to create a safe and conscious awareness of what is happening, without having to resort to unconscious primitive defenses to protect against overwhelming feelings. There are three clinical roles of containment in TSM:

1) the containing double,
2) the body double, and
3) the keeper of defenses.

The Containing Double (CD).   The containing double represents the part of self that brings unconditional acceptance. It is the archetypal good mother. It provides support no matter what level of distress. The CD helps put words onto unprocessed trauma material as it emerges in awareness to maintain a balance between affect and cognition. This role has been operationalized and tested as an intervention module to show that the CD significantly decreases dissociation with trauma survivors (Hudgins, Drucker, & Metcalf, 1998).

The team leader prescribes the containing double any time s/he assesses that the protagonist is starting to get overwhelmed emotionally or is using primitive defenses. The assistant leader can also assign auxiliaries to be a CD for any group member who is need of support. The CD speaks in first person and becomes a part of self for the client, who internalizes self-support as the words are spoken.

The TL prescribed the containing double for Vladamir since he stated he had trouble controlling his rage at home. When he was talking to the soul of his mother, he was directed to speak in his own language. While the CD could only speak English, the TAE used nonverbal doubling with words to provide containment. The CD followed the movements of the protagonist and when Vladamir started to fist his hands in rage, the CD opened and closed his hands repeatedly. He put words to what he was doing to interrupt the affective escalation: "I am so mad I feel like hitting out, but I can open and close my hands instead. I can decide how I want to express my anger." Vladamir could see this action and hear the words. He was able to take a deep breath, open and shut his fists, and regain better control of his rage in the present moment.

Body Double (BD).   This clinical role constantly keeps clients focused on healthy body awareness, even when triggered by body memories.

The body double enacts the cellular, nonverbal, intuitive, and emotional communication from the person's body to the mind. The body double is used to assist clients to develop a clearer communication relationship with their body in order to rebuild what has been termed "the body of trust" (Ridge, 1998).

The body double's purpose is to create a sense of safety and containment within the realm of the physical body. The TAE taking the body double role speaks in first person since it is a part of self. Often, the words are slow as the body is not used to speaking. The BD paces the words so that the client is not overwhelmed or triggered into primitive defenses. The body double also keeps a clear boundary within the protagonist, sometimes, reminding the group when some quiet time is needed to hear the body's messages.

On her evaluation form, Andrea stated, "The body double was the crucial intervention for me. Without that, I would still be anorexic and in love with my scales. Now, I can start liking my body again. Thank you."

Keeper of Defenses (KD).   This role is the third clinical role prescribed for containment in TSM. The containing double increases containment with feelings and thoughts. The body double contains body sensations and establishes a physical sense of vitality and spontaneity. The keeper of defenses is enacted to contain defenses.

The KD is the antidote for the automatic use of such primitive defenses as denial, dissociation, multiple states of consciousness, idealization, identification with the aggressor, and projective identification. This prescriptive role is further described in chapter 9 as part of the intervention module of the manager of healthy functioning, a transformative role.

Jim said that the keeper of defenses was a crucial prescriptive role for him as a recovering alcoholic. He was able to use Alcoholics Anonymous to get sober and to help him replace the defensive use of drugs and alcohol. The program, though, was not enough to work through flashbacks, body memories, and dissociation. In an individual TSM session, Jim was able to concretize a keeper of defenses that was a "timely and competent guard." The next time he experienced a flashback at home, he was able to guard against dissociation by calling a friend.

When the prescriptive roles are enacted, they define a state of spontaneous learning. When this state of new learning is generated, the change agent role emerges. This is the first transformative role and will be described later in this chapter.

TRAUMA-BASED ROLES

The trauma survivor's intrapsychic role atom also provides a clinical map of the internalization of traumatic experience. The second category of roles in the TSIRA, the trauma-based roles, include

- the holder of defenses,
- the defenses,
- the victim role,
- the perpetrator role, and
- the role of an abandoning authority.

The holder of defenses and the defenses themselves keep unprocessed trauma material locked in trauma bubbles. These trauma-based roles come about automatically to protect clients from being emotionally destroyed by the experience and serve the purpose of survival at the time of trauma. Victim, perpetrator, and abandoning authority roles represent the internalization of the experience of trauma. These trauma-based roles hold unprocessed information in state dependent trauma bubbles. Identifying, experiencing, and expressing the roles of victim, perpetrator, and abandoning authority tells the story of trauma, so developmental repair can occur.

As previously noted, trauma-based roles are only enacted after the prescriptive roles are established in order to prevent uncontrolled regression and unconscious abreaction. Even if a protagonist spontaneously sees his or her victim self or perpetrator figures on the stage, the team leader has a clinical responsibility to make sure the prescriptive roles are stabilized before further enactment of these trauma-based roles. This too is an element of TSM that differentiates it from classical psychodrama. The TL does not follow the protagonist, but rather s/he directs the drama clinically as needed for safety.

Holder of the Defenses

The role of holder of defenses evolved from my experience as team leader directing groups of trauma survivors. I would ask a protagonist to pick someone to concretize dissociation when it was interrupting a drama. What I found with that intervention was that both the protagonist and auxiliary then started dissociating!

A clinical role was created to control and hold the dissociation so that it could be used if chosen, but not happen automatically and unconsciously. As the holder role is enacted, clients experience their rigid use of defenses. They see that the defenses are really survival based, and not appropriate to the stresses of adult functioning.

As Jim began to set up a scene from his childhood, he started to dissociate and forgot for a moment where he was. He became very still and looked around in a dazed fashion. The auxiliaries in the prescriptive roles offered an anchor into positive states, but it was as if Jim had floated away and could not hear nor see them.

As team leader, I asked him to concretize the dissociation floating around the room. He picked up several white scarves and created a veil over his face. Then I asked him to pick someone to be his holder of defenses, so the dissociation could begin to be labeled. The holder role was charged with controlling the dissociation and being "on call" if it was needed during Jim's drama. Several times the holder brought the dissociation back in automatically. Each time Jim could say, "No, I don't need that right now," strengthening the keeper function of the emerging prescriptive role.

In the Therapeutic Spiral Model, all defenses are honored for the survival role they have played in the person's life. The "no shame, no blame" rule applies here, particularly for people who have struggled with addiction—whether to food, alcohol, drugs, sex, work, exercise, et cetera. TSM understands that defenses were needed in the past. In the present, the prescriptive roles create the space for defenses to be identified and used only as necessary.

Defenses

As noted in chapter 1, the experience of severe trauma overwhelms even the most healthily functioning person. When this happens, ego defenses are automatically engaged to prevent psychological death. The Therapeutic Spiral Model concretizes three levels of defensive roles:

1) primitive,
2) compulsive/addictive, and
3) maladaptive.

Primitive Defenses. Primitive defenses are the roles of last resort when trauma happens. They operate at an automatic level of self-protection.

They are survival mechanisms that defend against psychological annihilation at the time of trauma. Primitive defenses include, but are not limited to, dissociation, denial, multiple states of consciousness, idealization, projective identification, and identification with the aggressor (described in more detail in chapter 1).

In TSM, the defenses are concretized in the action so that they can be seen and observed in conscious awareness. Dissociation is a veil of white haze. Denial is a blindfold around eyes and ears. Projective identification becomes a ball passed between two people. Primitive defenses are enacted and made tangible to the therapeutic relationship for change.

Vladamir was able to identify that he was using denial to cope with the fear and belief that his sister and mother had been raped and murdered. He concretized denial by placing a black scarf around his eyes and saying, "I can't see what happened to them. I can't feel it if I can't see it. Maybe nothing happened to them." Slowly, he chose to take off the scarf of denial and to look consciously at the scene that haunted him—his mother and sister being violently dragged off by Bosnian soldiers. Then, he could find and release his dissociated rage and grief with the support and witnessing of his multicultural colleagues at the refugee center.

Obsessions, Compulsions, and Addictions.   This second set of defensive, trauma-based roles in the TSIRA form as primitive defenses become overused and ingrained in the personality structure. Defenses start to take over life when they become obsessions, compulsions, and addictions. In all cases, these efforts at compensation only push feelings further down and make it more likely that they will break through trauma bubbles in unpredictable ways.

Obsessions and compulsions often respond to medications to treat the disrupted neurobiological processes that happen from trauma. Many behaviors that become addictions clearly start off as defensive behaviors. Having a drink to relax at night, exercising to get fit, working late some nights, taking prescribed medicine for pain are ways people cope with their feelings. For trauma survivors however, there is a greater risk that they will abuse alcohol, drugs, and even healthy defenses like work and exercise. And often the abuse can become a pattern of addiction long after the trauma itself has stopped. For many people, 12-step programs are the first step in personal recovery from addiction.

Andrea was clearly caught in an obsessive-compulsive pattern of thinking about her weight and weighed herself over 100 times a day. When she would start to feel emotions linked to her rape or see the images of the boys' faces, she would unconsciously go over to the scales and weigh herself. This compulsion prevented her from regressing but it did not allow her to work through the unprocessed information in her trauma bubbles. She would get stuck in defending against her anxiety and repeat the pattern over and over of weighing herself, wasting hours a day in useless efforts of control. As she internalized the role of a body double for herself, Andrea was able to let go of her obsessions and compulsive behaviors around food, weight, and control. As the defenses of her eating disorder were modified, she experienced feelings of shame, loss, and rage, which she was able to express safely in TSM groups.

Maladaptive Roles. These trauma-based roles represent the higher order defenses. As people with PTSD gain more coping skills, maladaptive roles develop that are still defensive and rigid, but they are less disruptive to daily life. A few examples of these kinds of roles are the unnoticed caretaker, the controlling mother, the overachieving good girl, the adult-child, the committed rescuer, and so on.

Jim had overdeveloped his adult-child and rescuer roles as a way to feel better about himself. As head counselor at the halfway house, he could concentrate his energy on the "guys who just got out of treatment and need me." Like Andrea and her obsessive weighing, however, these maladaptive roles got in the way of him fully healing from his childhood abuse.

In a restoration and renewal drama, Jim was able to practice his rescuer role toward himself rather than using it only for other people. When he was working on his childhood trauma, the team leader asked him to "rescue yourself from your father. You know how to do that from your work with the guys. Use it now for yourself." Immediately, he moved into action and physically intervened in the scene to get his wounded child out of the trauma scene with his father.

Internalization of Trauma Roles

Clients easily understand this category of TSIRA roles from their personal experience with trauma. Trauma-based roles serve the function of communication. They hold the story of trauma, until it is safe to be processed. The TSM divides the internal representations of trauma into

- the victim role,
- the perpetrator role, and
- the role of an abandoning authority.

For many trauma survivors, either the victim or perpetrator role seems to have dominated their lives. They have been suicidal and murderous. They have acted out against themselves and others. The role that is often subtler is that of the abandoning authority.

People internalize self-abandonment and feel worthless and filled with shame when they cannot prevent trauma from happening. With PTSD, this leads to abandoning one's own authority for self in many ways. People neglect self-care. They repeat destructive relationships. They hide and isolate themselves from life.

Trauma-based roles are often enacted by trained members of an action trauma team to prevent retraumatization to clients. No client is ever role reversed into a victim or perpetrator role unless the prescriptive roles are fully developed. Even then, role reversal only happens with support through the containing double or the body double. (See chapter 10.)

Victim Role. This trauma-based role carries the state dependent experience of being overwhelmed and victimized by trauma. Enacting the role of victim can concretize many of the dissociated thoughts, feelings, images, and sensations held in trauma bubbles. The powerlessness, the helplessness, and despair of the traumatic experience is stored in this role. In the TSM, the TL uses the word victim to accurately label the victimization experience, and then quickly moves to label the role as the wounded child. In that way the vulnerabilities and wounds of the trauma experience can be accessed without shame or blame.

Wounded Child Role. In the TSM, the wounded child role takes victimization and portrays it more compassionately to engage the power of change in a drama. Often, a protagonist will respond to an auxiliary that is expressing the hurt, pain, and despair of the wounded child and begin to discriminate being a victim from the natural expression of trauma.

Andrea had unconsciously embraced the victim role following the gang rape. She gave up all activity, stayed at home, and spent all of her time obsessing about food until she was depressed, suicidal, and anorexic. Six months after her trauma, she remained stuck in a victim stance with little hope of change.

During her weekly TSM group, Andrea asked someone to play "her victim self." Ann, a TAE, took the role and enacted the feelings and behaviors that Andrea had shared over the past few weeks. She walked slowly, head down in shame. She said, "I am hopeless, nothing will ever change. My life is ruined." From the role of her "good mother," Andrea was able to make contact with this part of herself in a new way. She said,

> I see you are carrying all the shame from the rape. It was not your fault. It's true that you did drink too much and made yourself vulnerable. But you did not deserve what happened to you. Those 4 boys that raped you—the shame belongs to them, not to you. You are OK.

When she role reversed into her victim role with a body double by her side, Andrea was able to listen to what her good mother role said and she began to sob deeply. The following dialogue facilitated her healing and letting go of the victim role so she could experience herself as a survivor rather than a victim.

Body Double:　I can stay in my body while I listen to my good mother. I can feel my feet on the floor and feel my breath coming in and out of my mouth.

Andrea in victim role:　OK, I can listen . . . it is so good to hear that it is not my fault. I was so sure it was because I got drunk. I mean I did drink too much. I did.

Body Double:　Yes, I did drink too much. And right now I am not drunk. My body is alive. I am breathing. I can see the group around me. I can let go of the shame.

Andrea in victim role:　[Starts to sob] I want to let go of the shame . . . I do . . . I do . . . it is killing me. I hate my body so much I just want it to die.

Good mother:　Andrea, Andrea, come here and let me hold you. You didn't deserve what those boys did no matter whether you were drunk or not. You are not to blame for their actions. They were wrong. Please, please believe me. You are a good person. Your body is good.

Body Double:　Yes, my body is good. Today, it is no longer physically injured. I can feel my ability to walk, to move, to look at people. Today, my body is healing.

Andrea as victim role begins to shift:　OK, today my body is OK. I can even see that the shame I have been carrying around does not belong to me. I can feel ashamed for getting drunk. But I do not have to take the shame that the rapes were my fault. I can be more gentle with myself, my wounded child self.

Perpetrator Role.   This trauma-based role holds the internalization of the violence that was experienced by the self during trauma. The perpetrator role carries the self-hate, self-criticism, and urge to act out violently toward self or others. This internalized role can even result in suicide attempts or murderous intent toward others.

The perpetrator role also holds the power of the trauma survivor. Like the victim role, the perpetrator role holds state dependent learning. Thus, it needs to be encountered during TSM work, but only after the prescriptive roles are stabilized.

Vladamir found himself enacting the perpetrator role internally. He told himself that he was "no good" because he had not been able to rescue his mother and sister, despite being held down on the ground by five other men. He blamed himself for being just like his captors and could not discriminate between them and himself when he first started training in the TSM.

An important drama for Vladamir was his interaction with an auxiliary in the role of the soul of his mother. She showed him forgiveness and understanding. Only then could he let go of the internalized perpetrator role that was destroying his own life. She said,

> Of course I wanted you to survive, to live. That was what mattered to me . . . that my son survived. Please do not feel guilty. You did the best you could. I know that. If there was anything to forgive I would give you forgiveness, but there is no need for that. You did what I wanted. You survived. I love you.

The Abandoning Authority Role.   This TSM trauma-based role is internalized from the experience of having no one to rescue or care for the protagonist at the time of trauma. This role of abandonment is then enacted toward self in relation to boundaries, safety, and empowerment. It is also repeated toward others in terms of parenting, teaching, and other authority roles.

The role of the abandoning authority may be the parent that did not intervene, but can also represent school, church, or a government that did not provide safety and help. Often the abandoning authority role needs to be changed before either of the other trauma-based roles can be addressed. People must accept authority for their own lives to change.

In a workshop, Tricia said she wanted to "take my own authority and stop the screams of my 5-year-old." The team leader asked her to set up the stuck image of herself screaming and screaming as a 5-year-old child. She described a scene with her godfather that happened when she was 5 years old. In this scene, she states that they were in the barn when he physically backed her up against a stall where some baby calves lived. Then he forced her to perform oral sex on him, left her there, and walked off.

As she witnesses this trauma-based scene and starts to feel powerless, the TL asks her in her adult role, "Where is your authority to save this child?" She says she does not know and begins to cry. He directs her to "create an authority from the group and see how you can get some help to stop the screaming."

The trauma-based scene freezes on the stage, while Tricia creates "a spirit of compassion" with three group members. Vladamir is picked to play "powerful compassion." Andrea is covered with yellow scarves and is called "bright light." Jim's role, which stands behind the other two, is "action change" and is concretized as a glowing spirit.

Tricia role reverses and becomes her glowing spirit. She grabs the hands of her bright light and powerful compassion and rescues her screaming 5-year-old. She says, "You are my angel. I love you. Do not scream now. You are safe with me. I will take care of you." The spirit of compassion offers comfort to the screams of the child.

Usually, a TSM drama explores one of the trauma-based roles at a time. This structure provide a sense of boundaries and containment. When the trauma-based roles interact with the prescriptive roles, they provide new narrative labeling for unprocessed trauma bubbles. When structured for clinical containment, these same roles can access conscious reexperiencing and chosen abreaction of unconscious trauma material.

TRANSFORMATIVE ROLES

The third category of roles in the TSIRA is the transformative role. When prescriptive roles are enacted with the trauma-based roles, the energy of new spontaneity and creativity is added. New individualized roles emerge, named the transformative roles in the Therapeutic Spiral Model.

There are three psychological functions that new transformative roles serve for healthy functioning:

1) autonomy,
2) connection with others, and
3) integration.

Given that these roles are unique to each individual it is hard to provide all encompassing categories of enactment. It often appears that transformative roles include at least one of the following, however: the sleeping-awakening child, a change agent, manager of healthy functioning, a good enough mother or father, and/or a good enough God.

The Sleeping-Awakening Child

This transformative role seems to be a very important one for trauma survivors. As described by Sheridan and Hudgins (1990), this transformative role contains all the natural talents, gifts, and potential of a person's life. When trauma happens, defenses push down not only the trauma material but also the best parts of self to survive. This role helps access the undamaged part of self by enacting the sleeping-awakening child.

When introduced, this transformative role is often seen as a child role, even a baby. As energy and time for experiencing are given to facilitate the sleeping-awakening child, the role begins to develop. The same qualities of potential, talent, and natural skill move from being a nascent possibility in a child role to full creative enactment in an adult form.

Jim was aware of the concept of being an adult child of an alcoholic. He had read about his inner child. But whenever he went to get in touch with that part of self, all he found was the experience of wounding, pain, and trauma. During one session, we worked to concretize a sleeping child that was "waiting for you to make the world safe enough today so that I can be all that I was meant to be." As he developed this role, he found that he was much more creative and involved with the recovering addicts in the halfway house. He discovered that he had quite a talent for leadership and was able to establish a new group for "his guys" that focused on finding the "happy, joyous, and free" in recovery.

The Change Agent Role

The change agent role is a unique embodiment of a client's personal experience of the state of spontaneity and creativity. This role encompasses the functions of restoration, containment, and observation, but is more than the sum total of the individual prescriptive roles. The change agent emerges spontaneously from the interaction of prescriptive roles with trauma-based patterns and signals the end of Scene 1 in the TSM. The change agent is seen as a significant turning point in healing self-organization. This role is the antidote to the internalization of the abandoning authority role that comes from trauma.

The change agent must be identified and incorporated into a TSM drama before consciously reexperiencing trauma-based roles. Often clients demonstrate the ability to rescue themselves by stopping old patterns. If the protagonist is frozen in the drama, unable to protect a child role, a group member can spontaneously respond with a change agent role through projective identification. S/he may stand up and scream "stop," rush in and rescue the child from the perpetrator, or nudge the protagonist to do so.

For Andrea, the change agent role that made a difference for her came about when she was able to access her "righteous rage" toward the boys who raped her. In a drama she was able to express to them her hatred, rage, and grief for what they had done to her innocence. Only then could she evolve beyond the victim role she was stuck in.

Manager of Healthy Functioning (MHF)

The manager of healthy functioning role is generated through the interaction of the prescriptive role of the keeper of defenses and the trauma-based holder of the defenses role. When spontaneity and creativity are added, the manager of healthy function develops.

This role allows the protagonist to stay present in the moment through adaptive responses such as self-support and connections to others. Primitive defenses and obsessions, compulsions, and addictions are not needed. Life can be lived from a view of healthy here and now functioning without defensive maneuvering.

CONCLUSIONS

This chapter and the following show the importance of the trauma survivor's intrapsychic role atom in the Therapeutic Spiral Model. It clinically guides the enactment of all roles to create safety and prevent uncontrolled regression with experiential methods. Prescriptive roles complete pre-trauma work to build up ego strength and adaptive capacity. Next, the TSIRA provides both client and therapist with an outline, a clinical structure for the internalization of trauma-based roles. Victim, perpetrator, and abandoning authority roles have been defined and will be demonstrated in action in later chapters. Defenses can be enacted to be used as needed.

Out of the spontaneous interaction between auxiliaries playing the prescriptive and trauma-based roles, new transformative roles emerge. These roles are individually created and based on promoting autonomy, connections to others, and a sense of spirituality. There are many ways that the TSIRA can be used in individual therapy, group sessions, and workshops. Clients are asked to write, draw, mold—create their TSIRA roles throughout a TSM workshop using markers, glitter, clay, sandtrays, etc.

This art project, using the TSIRA, as a guide, teaches clients the importance of building up restorative roles before they put the trauma-based roles on their project. Roles of restoration, observation, and containment are always put on the representation of the TSIRA first to mark positive roles. For the first time, many people really recognize the impact of trauma in their lives when a beautiful mask, or sandtray, or soulprint body drawing is physically crushed, altered, or ripped as they add the internalized roles of victim, perpetrator, abandoning authority and defenses to their project. Relief is felt as the transformative roles emerge from the TSIRA whether on paper, in an art project or enacted on the stage.

The TSIRA is also very useful in individual experiential psychotherapy. When a trauma survivor first begins therapy, the clinician can ask them to draw their role atom using circles for the different roles. This can be used for initial assessment and then as a guide throughout therapy. You teach what the prescriptive roles are and ask the client to mark them on a paper if they have them. Then you ask them to mark their trauma-based roles. Look to see what roles are represented as smaller or larger than others are. How close or far away are the roles from the client's place in the center of the paper?

Like the visual images of the spiral and trauma bubbles, the TSIRA provides a link between the cognitive and experiential aspects of the TSM. Because it can be concretized in many forms combining words and actions, it allows the client to access some unprocessed information, while at the same time finding the labels to describe it according to role theory. This tool alone can guide safe experiential practice with trauma survivors.

CHAPTER SIX

Types of Conscious Reexperiencing Dramas for Developmental Repair

CHAPTER OVERVIEW

This chapter describes the fourth clinical action structure developed in the Therapeutic Spiral Model: the types of reexperiencing dramas (Hudgins, 1993; Hudgins, 2000). Each type of TSM drama is detailed with a session contract, clinical goals, and shared examples from clients. There are six types of reexperiencing dramas in TSM:

1) Restoration and Renewal
2) Dreams and Metaphors
3) Initial Discovery and Accurate Labeling
4) Uncovering and Exploring Core Trauma
5) Conscious Reexperiencing With Developmental Repair
6) Release and Transformation

Although these dramas are listed in a certain sequence, they need not proceed in this linear fashion. The type of drama contracted for between protagonist and team leader is determined by the clinical needs for safety. For example, when the TL assesses a need for ego-building, s/he contracts with the protagonist for a restoration and renewal drama. This type of drama targets increased experiencing of personal, interpersonal, and transpersonal resources as the clinical goal.

Contracting for an initial discovery and accurate labeling drama requires that the protagonist have the capacity to witness the enactment of traumatic material without decompensation. Conscious reexperiencing with developmental repair is designated only when intrapsychic structures and modified defenses support this deepest level of experiential practice.

PRIMARY PROCESS: THE TIME AND PLACE OF TSM DRAMAS

When first witnessing dramas in work with the Therapeutic Spiral Model, they can appear quite chaotic. After all, TSM dramas externalize the internal world of trauma survivors—with its attendant fragmented sensorimotor representations and intense dissociated feelings. Participants invariably question where and when the scene is anchored. What I explain is that when working with a "TSM trauma drama," the scene is set in primary process. Within the circle of safe experiencing, TSM concretizes the unprocessed fragments of trauma as they are stored, in trauma bubbles as primary process sensations, perceptions, smells, sounds, and tastes. This is primary process—the experience of internal processes without cognitive labels. In the TSM, the workings of the brain are literally externalized on the stage, so the protagonist can see the free associations, the blurred self and object relations, the dissociated images and feelings in order to make sense of them in the present.

When words become attached to primary process experience, it signifies that the unprocessed trauma material stored in the emotional centers of the brain is now accessible to the frontal cortex and higher order thinking processes. This is called secondary process thinking, when you are able to put words to your experiences, and is the goal of all psychotherapies, whether experiential or not.

Clinical contracts guide the protagonist, group, and team through the affect bridges, triggered associations, and primitive defenses for self-protection. This fourth TSM clinical action structure shows how to gently spiral into unprocessed trauma bubbles, rather than popping them open unpredictably.

CLINICAL CONTRACT WITH PROTAGONIST

A clinical, or session, contract with a protagonist is an essential feature to provide safety in the TSM. The stated contract gives the team an opportunity to plan ahead for clinical interventions for defenses, intense affect, and ego-state changes. It sets the structures in motion that promote regression in service of the ego. The contract supports reexperiencing in a conscious and chosen manner.

The session contract always addresses the following areas:

1)   The team leader or therapist contracts with the protagonist for the type of reexperiencing drama that is to be completed in the specific session.

2)   The team leader tells both the protagonist and group that they need not take any role that is uncomfortable. Knowing that the TAEs are trained specifically for this makes saying no easier for group members.

3)   The TL explains that there is no violent or sexual touching that happens with experiential methods. All touching, such as hands on the shoulder for action sociograms, is done with fully informed consent, and the right to say no.

4)   The TL explains that confidentiality is paramount for trauma survivors. No one is to tell who the protagonist is, but as important, no one is to share the protagonist's story, as even that can break confidentiality, without using names. Remember the stories that are shared are often the most private, unspeakable moments. Confidentiality needs to be stressed.

Once determined, this contract is stated aloud by the team leader and protagonist so that group members, the assistant leader, and the TAEs are all in agreement about the action that will follow. That way they can work together clinically to use experiential interventions in the service of the clients.

TYPES OF CONSCIOUS REEXPERIENCING DRAMAS

This chapter now defines the types of conscious reexperiencing dramas that were developed to further ensure a sense of clinical guidance, clear boundaries, and regression in the service of the ego in the Therapeutic Spiral Model.

RESTORATION AND RENEWAL

The first type of drama in TSM focuses on accessing, experiencing, and stabilizing a reliable and steady sense of personal and collective spontaneity, creativity, and spirituality. Restoration and renewal dramas build the energy needed to heal the depletion of body, mind, emotions, and spirit that is part of trauma. Before any other work can be done, basic self-organization must be energized, restored, and renewed for here and now functioning.

The Session Contract

In a restoration and renewal drama, the team leader contracts with the protagonist for a TSM drama that enacts prescriptive roles that are energizing to self-organization. Restorative roles of strength are always concretized. Enactment may also include roles of containment and observation as needed to build the healing state of spontaneity. A change agent role may appear as well.

Clinical Goals

A major clinical goal is to establish the state of spontaneous learning with the protagonist. Through on-going process assessment, the TL decides which prescriptive roles need to be enacted for this particular drama. They are put into action and the protagonist role reverses as needed to increase positive experiencing.

Clinically, there are three stages in therapy where a restoration and renewal drama is indicated:

1) at the beginning of experiential treatment to increase energy and build spontaneity;
2) during the therapeutic process to refuel the energy reserves while uncovering and exploring core trauma material; and
3) at the end of therapy to celebrate transformative roles and self-integration.

While restoration is necessary before any trauma-based roles are experienced, a renewal drama can also be a refresher from the intense abreactive work of conscious reexperiencing of core trauma material. The roles that were created at the beginning of therapy to build spontaneity, creativity, and spirituality can be accessed again and again to support active experiencing of past and present in a balanced learning state.

During one Surviving Spirits workshop, Tricia contracted to "enact all the significant female roles" that had given her a sense of self-esteem, personal power, and professional identity in her life. This developmental drama gave her a deeply felt sense of generational restoration and a confidence in herself that she had not experienced for a long time. New transgenerational messages flowed through to Tricia. Stoic Great Grandmother said, "I see how you have become a powerful attorney and carried on our matriarchal line of power. I am proud of you." Loving Aunt Dorothy, her father's sister, said, "I have not always understood you, but I have always loved you. It was a pleasure to watch you grow up into such a fine woman." Her surprising second grade teacher, Mrs. Murphy, said, "You are one of the brightest students I have ever had. I am glad to see you are using your mind to sort out your truth. You will go far with your mind and your heart in connection." Her supportive best friend, Kathy, said, "I will always love you as a chosen sister. You are one of the kindest and most generous women I have ever met. You mean the world to me."

When these restorative roles are actively experienced they provide healing mentally, emotionally, interpersonally, and spiritually for people with PTSD.

Team Roles

During a restoration and renewal drama, the teams takes on prescriptive roles as requested by the protagonist or TL. The AL monitors the group and assigns containing doubles or other supportive roles as needed. The TAES are active in collecting information from group members and bringing it to the AL for spontaneous and creative action.

DREAMS AND METAPHORS

Classical psychodrama has long enacted dreams and metaphors. In the TSM, dreams, myths, symbols, fairy tales, and metaphors can be enacted to explore the richness of unconscious representations of trauma. This type of TSM drama is frequently used in community settings as a safe way to share about common trauma without a great deal of personal self-disclosure.

A contract for dreams and metaphors gives the team a chance to assess the level of spontaneity, ego strength, and interpersonal support available to the protagonist—before going into deeper levels of experiencing trauma bubbles. Sometimes these metaphoric journeys are used as a warm-up for deeper uncovering and exploring of dramas. Often, the entire session is used to portray a single dream or concretize a favorite childhood myth to increase spontaneity.

The Session Contract

When the protagonist contracts to enact a dream or metaphor, it is important to keep the enactment at the level of symbolic representation. Relying on this clinical contract for a meaning making structure maintains a level of safety for the protagonist and group. If trauma-based fragments do intrude on the abstract enactment, the director consciously addresses this with the protagonist, and either contracts for another type of drama or uses action interventions to strengthen the boundaries on the primary process material.

Clinical Goals

The clinical goal with dreams and metaphors is to explore unconscious representations of trauma, and to keep the boundaries on the enactment to this abstract level. With this contract, the protagonist can experience the prescriptive and transformative roles, as well as hints of the trauma-based ones, without being triggered into uncontrolled regression.

Jim had kept a dream journal for years in the hopes that "it would stop the nightmares." In a weekend workshop, he contracted to enact a fragment of a recurring dream. In this dream, he was pursued by wolves until he was backed up against a tree and about to be killed. Then he would wake up, bathed in sweat.

The TL directed Jim to pick group members to play prescriptive roles for him. He chose "the spirit of Mother Earth," "a ferocious bear," and "a watchful owl." Thus, he populated his primary process world with positive roles to support exploration into unconscious symbols.

When he had team members play the howling, snarling, raging wolves in the psychodrama, Jim was able to summon up his bear to fight them off—after owl had alerted him to their presence in time. The final scene of the dream was being held in the arms of the spirit of Mother Earth, in the hopes that the nightmares would stop.

After this drama, Jim reported being free of nightmares for the most part. When he did have the occasional nightmare, he could now summon up the experience of Mother Earth comforting him and go gently back to sleep.

Team Roles

The Team Leader uses interventions to support containment and to increase spontaneity, not to go into unconscious material behind the symbols. Trained auxiliaries know just how to play shadow roles in dreams and metaphors, so that they do not trigger personal trauma responses in the protagonist or group. When someone is triggered, they are invaluable in providing support and containment. The AL keeps a close eye on everyone to help maintain a sense of creativity and play.

INITIAL DISCOVERY AND ACCURATE LABELING

All experiential psychotherapies label thoughts, feelings, and behaviors based on the bodily felt sense of the experience, rather than on internalized representations. The TSM delineates a type of drama, called initial discovery and accurate labeling of trauma. It concretizes consciously remembered experiences for the purpose of observation and corrective narrative labels. It takes the bodily felt sense of a known trauma and connects it to new meanings in the present.

The structure of this type of drama supports cognitive interventions into the experiential state dependent learning from the past. The protagonist revisits past scenes in action with the clinical focus on meaning making. As always, prescriptive roles are experienced so that trauma-based scenes are contained and can be observed. At the end of an accurate labeling drama, a transformative role—the change agent—emerges, that can identify and interrupt old trauma patterns.

This type of TSM drama is indicated prior to exploring unprocessed trauma material to provide a cognitive container for dissociated trauma bubbles. It can also be useful to the client to contract for an accurate labeling drama after they have, in fact, uncovered significant new sensorimotor representations that need to be integrated into meaning structures.

The Session Contract

The clinical contract for a TSM drama of initial discovery and accurate labeling is to enact remembered memories, fragments, feelings, and behaviors. The contract is to connect them with accurate narrative meanings based on the client's active experiencing in the present. The contract is not for emotional expression, but for the emergence of experiential meaning from one's own experience.

Often, dissociated affects are triggered during an accurate labeling drama. When this happens, the clinical contract calls for containment, not expression of affect. Role reversing the client into prescriptive roles of observation (OE, client role) provides the antidote to intrusive feelings, and puts the emphasis back on meaning making. This is another distinction from classical psychodrama. TSM does not follow the affect until there is a balanced state of cognitive awareness.

Clinical Goals

The clinical goal is to find accurate, narrative labels that emerge out of personal experiencing. This is most often accomplished by concretizing conscious fragments of memory from trauma bubbles, with the support of the prescriptive roles. The protagonist then watches and observes trauma scenes with intense affects held by TAEs. Brief role reversals into trauma-based roles may provide additional information, but the protagonist does not stay in these roles for long in this type of drama.

The clinical goal is to have the prescriptive and trauma-based roles interact until a transformative change agent role emerges from the spontaneity of the moment. This transformative role shows the protagonist's ability to spiral into trauma bubbles and then spiral back up with new meanings. It is an indication that clients are ready to go deeper into unprocessed material in another drama.

Tricia contracted for an accurate labeling drama during her individual therapy when Ann was there as a trained auxiliary ego. In the safety of this setting, she was able to describe several scenes of sexual abuse from her father and godfather. She had always had a visual fragment of the terror on her face the first time her father forced oral sex when she was 3 years old.

When the trained auxiliary ego walked through the actions of these scenes, Andrea witnessed her own narrative from her OE role. She was able, for the first time, to truly understand that the sexual contact with her father had, in fact, been abuse and not "Daddy's love." This was a profound insight that was instrumental in ridding her current sexual relationship with her husband of transferential intrusions. Out of this insight, Andrea consciously created the transformative role of "the clear thinker" and added it to her increasing role repertoire for healthy functioning. The clear thinker became the change agent to help her accurately label abuse, an important step in her healing.

Team Roles

As clinicians, team members neither influence nor validate the protagonist's meanings. The team's professional view is that this is the client's memory, the client's experience, and he or she must find the labels that fit. During TSM dramas that are contracted to explore conscious memories for accurate meaning, the team's auxiliary work should replicate the protagonist's experience as closely as possible.

UNCOVERING AND EXPLORING CORE TRAUMA

Many protagonists report chronic symptoms of PTSD even after initial discovery and accurate labeling of traumatic experiences has been achieved. In fact, many clients begin experiential treatment in the Therapeutic Spiral Model at this point in their recovery from trauma. Cognitive insight is established and ego strength is in place; however, they are still haunted by intrusive sensory, perceptual, emotional, and behavioral symptoms.

In the uncovering and exploring of core trauma, the protagonist contracts to explore unprocessed material contained in trauma bubbles. The purpose of consciously experiencing and expressing fragmented trauma images and dissociated emotions is to make new life-affirming meanings out of past experiences. After the prescriptive roles are concretized and the transformative change agent role has been generated, a protagonist can safely contract to uncover and explore core trauma memories. In this type of drama, the team leader and protagonist explore the unprocessed primary process representations stored in trauma bubbles.

The affective management structures and advanced intervention modules (see chapter 9) of TSM promote controlled regression. Chosen, conscious, supported regression allows protagonists to experience state dependent roles such as victim and perpetrator safely. They are not overwhelmed with affect, but able to stay conscious and keep their cognitive processes intact in the present.

The Session Contract

When a protagonist has demonstrated use of the change agent role to prevent uncontrolled regression, s/he is ready to contract for a drama that uncovers and explores unconscious trauma bubbles. The clinical contract is to use the prescriptive and transformative roles to hold unprocessed trauma material in conscious awareness for further exploration without triggering primitive defenses. The contract is for controlled regression into trauma-based roles.

Clinical Goals

The clinical goal of an uncovering and exploring TSM drama is to access, consciously reexperience, express, and work through unconscious elements of a core trauma scene. This is done for the purpose of memory retrieval, emotional processing, and integration of the experience into current information processing systems. The clinical goal is to support controlled regression and conscious abreaction of dissociated feelings. By directly accessing the unprocessed information stored in the emotional centers of the brain in a conscious exploration, new labels emerge to make sense out of traumatic experiences.

Vladimir contracted to do a drama to uncover and explore his fears about what had happened to his mother and sisters. For many months, he had tried to deny or control his fears that they were raped and murdered. Obsessive thoughts tried to keep this out of awareness, but images and feelings kept intruding on him when he was trying to do his paperwork at the refugee center, or sitting home alone late at night.

He set up prescriptive roles in Scene 1. Then he told the group what he thought had happened to his family. They were raped by the soldiers. Maybe they made his mother watch as his sisters were killed first. They were all shot and pushed in a joint grave.

This trauma-based scene was put into action with Peter (TAE) representing a group of soldiers by using empty chairs to make the larger perpetrator role. Ann (TAE) enacted one of his sisters while Andrea played the other with the support of a containing double. His mother was portrayed by Colette, another TAE. Jim spontaneously jumped up and took on the role of energetic protector, joining Vladimir in his efforts. This time, in surplus reality, they could stop the soldiers from taking away his family. Together, they surrounded the soldiers and he said,

> This has to stop. Please . . . just months ago we were friends, neighbors. Stop and think what you are doing. This is my mother. This is my sister. You have mothers and sisters. How would you want them to be treated?

The team leader briefly role reversed Vladimir into the perpetrator role held by Peter to see if, in fact, the soldiers had listened. The words of confrontation were repeated by Jim, who stepped into the client role. With Peter beside him as a containing double for the perpetrator role, Vladimir found he did listen. He laid down his gun and started to cry.

The team leader reversed Vladimir back to his role as protagonist. Peter enacted the scene of remorse and change by the soldiers. In this uncovering and exploring of his fears around the rape and murder of his family, Vladimir was able to experience developmental repair. He could not stop the abduction in real life, but in a TSM drama, he could confront the soldiers and bring back their humanity. He had a new experience to replace the old obsessive images of his rupture from his family.

Team Roles

The use of an action trauma team is especially necessary for clinical safety when conducting the uncovering and exploring of core trauma locked in trauma bubbles. When the protagonist moves into unconscious awareness, so do other group members. Projective identifications begin to fly around the room and are picked up unconsciously by other group members. Trauma bubbles can burst as participants become triggered by trauma scenes similar to their own.

The assistant leader and trained auxiliary egos support the maximum expansion of spontaneity for the protagonist and group members, while also providing a safe container for dissociated material and intense affects to arise. Therapists who must conduct groups alone can teach group members to work as a team to support each other in the processes of containment and expansion (Baratka, 1994).

Conscious Reexperiencing With Developmental Repair

The Therapeutic Spiral Model allows the protagonist full conscious reexperiencing of what happened and the complete expression of his or her response to the trauma in action. When clinically indicated, clients contract for conscious reexperiencing of a traumatic memory from all roles, including victim and perpetrator. The TSM intervention module for the safe enactment of these trauma-based roles is presented in chapter 10.

These dramas are enacted for the purpose of developmental repair. The state dependent learning that was frozen at the time of core trauma is enlivened with the energy of spontaneity, creativity, and healing. Following the principles of conscious reexperiencing (see chapters 7 and 8), the protagonist experiences controlled regression into trauma-based roles and unprocessed memories safely.

Each conscious reexperiencing TSM drama follows a clearly deline-ated clinical action structure: the principles of conscious reexperiencing with developmental repair (see chapters 7 and 8). After concretizing the prescriptive and transformative roles, the protagonist talks, observes, witnesses, reenacts, reexperiences, and repairs core trauma scenes in action.

The final scene in all conscious reexperiencing dramas is always one of developmental repair. Through the use of surplus reality, the protagonist finds new solutions to old trauma patterns. The past can stop repeating itself.

The Session Contract

The clinical contract is to follow the principles of conscious reexperienc-ing to guide controlled regression into trauma-based roles. Then, victim and perpetrator roles can be consciously reexperienced within the safety of the container of the prescriptive/transformative roles, affective man-agement structures, and team support. Most importantly, the contract includes and emphasizes the goal of developmental repair in order that the cathartic abreaction be truly therapeutic and to prevent re-traumatization. Chapters 7 and 8 detail an entire conscious reexperiencing drama of a childhood sexual abuse scene for illustration of this type of drama. Detailed here are the clinical steps that guide directing decisions during TSM conscious reexperiencing dramas.

Step 1. In Scene 1 of all TSM dramas, the protagonist consciously builds the prescriptive roles needed to unlock, retrieve, experience, and express unconscious material stored in trauma bubbles. This ensures that the protagonist has the containing double, the observing ego, and the client role available as needed during conscious reexperiencing.

Step 2. In Scene 2, the trauma scene is enacted (often by TAEs) following the TSM principles of conscious reexperiencing. The protagonist talks about, observes, and witnesses the trauma scene to make sure that s/he can stay present and in a state of spontaneous learning. Often, the team members take the manager of healthy functioning role during the initial presentation of a trauma scene to help the protagonist and group members to modify their defenses. At the end of Scene 2, defenses have been contained and a change agent has emerged. Only then, can one safely move to conscious reexperiencing of trauma-based roles.

Step 3. Additional trauma-based scenes of controlled regression into the victim or perpetrator roles are experienced by the protagonist with the support of the prescriptive roles. This may consist of one or more scenes, depending on the time available and team support possible. The principles of conscious reexperiencing guide controlled regression and chosen expression of long-dissociated feelings. The intervention module for the safe enactment of trauma-based roles is fully utilized. (See chapters 7–10 for demonstration and processing.)

Step 4. The final scene, one of developmental repair, is achieved in this type of drama by the use of surplus reality scenes. The protagonist can enact and experience the longed for object relations with self and others. New life-affirming endings of personal autonomy and integration are experienced. Connections to others and to a sense of universal meaning build and develop in any repair scene the protagonist chooses to experience.

Surplus reality endings, however, must be consistent with the protagonist's set of introjected internal object relations. When these developmental repair scenes are so structured, the self actually experiences the surplus reality of what "should have been" in the past and what is now possible to be experienced in the present.

Clinical Goals

The clinical goal in this type of TSM drama is to consciously reexperience trauma-based roles to access state dependent learning. Dissociated feelings are expressed and integrated into new meaning structures. Developmental repair happens. This level of TSM drama produces profound healing, thanks to the use of an action trauma team to prevent retraumatization (see chapters 7 and 8 for demonstration of a conscious reexperiencing drama with developmental repair).

Team Roles

The team leader and action trauma team stage the action of the conscious reexperiencing drama with care and clinical concern. Both the protagonist and the group are guided to consciously spiral to the depths of reexperiencing trauma based roles. TAEs often take the victim and perpetrator roles. They know how to walk the edge of increased experiencing without triggering primitive defenses. When a protagonist is ready they provide support for increased experiencing of his or her own trauma-based roles. Clients get to work at their own pace with clinical support.

Many times after a drama of conscious reexperiencing, team members are left with their own reactivation of trauma material and defenses. This is when the team meetings, described in chapter 11, provide a refuge for their own developmental repair, instead of increasing the risk of secondary posttraumatic stress disorder.

RELEASE AND TRANSFORMATION

The progression of the spiral image, from the energy of restoration to the deep experiencing of unprocessed trauma material, cycles back to dramas of release and transformation. While conscious reexperiencing and developmental repair can create experiential shifts in the boundaries of trauma bubbles and self-organization, these changes must be narratively labeled to be fully integrated. Dramas to release old roles and experience the new roles of transformation are alive with the energy and possibility of healing.

The Session Contract

The contract for a TSM drama of letting go and transformation is to release old trauma-based roles, and to develop new transformative roles. This contract is specifically about what role, what part of self, is to be released and transformed, as part of the healing process.

In a release and transformation drama, future projection is the most often used surplus reality intervention. As old trauma-based roles are let go, new roles need to be anchored in time and space. They can be practiced in the safety of a TSM drama prior to trying out the new roles in life. Alternatively, scenes can be set in the interpersonal reality of the group and used for role testing in the TSM session. Either way, the transformative possibilities of the future can be experienced in the here and now, and then used to draw the protagonist forward into new life meanings.

Clinical Goals

The clinical goal of a letting go and transformation drama is to anchor in new transformative roles and narrative labels. This is an opportunity to develop personal transformative roles of the sleeping-awakening child, the change agent, the manager of healthy functioning, good enough others, and spirituality.

This type of TSM drama can be contracted for at any point in the recovery process. It is often a good warm-up to deeper dramas. It can be a chance for practicing transformative roles. It is a wonderful type of drama to celebrate success.

Andrea contracted for a drama for letting go and transformation in an individual therapy session near the end of her TSM treatment. Using scarves, empty chairs, and objects in the room, she set up a transformative role scene. With the protection of her own powerful male energy (a bold red scarf) and the female energy of her best friend (empty chair draped in teal) by her side, Andrea was able to make a connection with the surplus reality image of a loving man in her future. She let go of her fears and her old labels of being ugly, no good, and evil.

With new innocence, Andrea looked this man in the face (an empty chair with a top hat on it). She was open, trusting, and yet not naïve. She truly experienced her transformation from a person suffering from anorexia and PTSD into an alive and vital young woman again.

Team Roles

During a letting go and transformation drama, the team is charged only with maximizing spontaneity. They may encourage, cajole, and place action demands on the protagonist and group to trust themselves in the moment, or to try out new behaviors, or to make new connections. These are the moments the action trauma team can sit back and enjoy good work done!

CONCLUSIONS

Chapter 6 has detailed the types of dramas in the Therapeutic Spiral Model. Each type has certain boundaries agreed upon in a clinical contract. Goals are set and clinical action structures followed. This is a major contribution of TSM to classical psychodrama and the clinical direction of people with PTSD.

TSM provides this clinical action structure to make sure that the seduction of trauma material does not push the trauma survivor into overexposure. Clinical contracts, boundaries of the drama, and clinical goals guide the enactment of each type of drama, so that there are no surprises for the protagonist or group. As shown in the last example, these TSM dramas can also be done in individual settings with the use of props to hold roles.

PART THREE

The Therapeutic Spiral Model in Action

Part III demonstrates the richness of the Therapeutic Spiral Model as it details a drama of conscious reexperiencing with developmental repair. Tricia shares her drama of childhood sexual abuse, showing the principles of conscious reexperiencing that guide the drama to the deepest levels of psychological healing. As TSM is an experiential method of learning, her drama is presented in full with actual dialogue adapted from videotapes of a *Surviving Spirits* workshop (Hudgins, 1993).

Only after the reader has experienced the drama, is it processed. In a parallel process to the protagonist, the reader will feel, see, and hear Tricia as she spirals into a past of childhood sexual abuse to emerge victorious at the end. Then, words will be put to the experience.

Chapters 7 and 8 present the actual drama of conscious reexperiencing with developmental repair. Chapter 7 reports Scenes 1 and 2, which build the prescriptive roles and modify primitive defenses. Chapter 8 follows Tricia as she uses controlled regression to actively experience two trauma memories in Scenes 3–5. Scene 6 completes the drama with developmental repair and true creative healing.

Then, chapters 9 and 10 process the drama and present the 14 advanced action intervention modules of TSM. Together they complete the clinical action structures that modify classical psychodrama for safe and effective use with PTSD and other stress-induced difficulties.

Principles of Conscious Reexperiencing With Developmental Repair: Scenes 1 and 2

CHAPTER OVERVIEW

The principles of conscious reexperiencing with developmental repair were developed to guide controlled regression and conscious abreaction. This clinical action structure, the fifth in the therapeutic spiral model, details the steps to increase active experiencing with trauma-based roles (Hudgins, 1993). When followed, these principles implement a series of six clear clinical decision points to support containment and conscious reexperiencing:

1) Talk
2) Observe
3) Witness
4) Reenact
5) Reexperience
6) Repair

These principles of conscious reexperiencing provide a clinical sequence of action interventions that ensures narrative labels are available at all times to guide regression in the service of the ego.

After presenting each principle, this chapter and the next follow Tricia in a TSM drama of conscious reexperiencing with developmental repair. Chapter 7 now details the structure provided by talking, observing, and witnessing, which are the three preliminary steps to conscious reexperiencing. Scenes 1 and 2 are presented with clinical dialogue and team interventions.

109

TALK

The first TSM principle of conscious reexperiencing is to verbally describe the trauma scenes that will be enacted. The protagonist tells the group what they will see enacted ahead of time. This verbal account allows the team to assess adaptive capacity, and to make TSM interventions for containment prior to the use of any experiential methods. In this way, talking enables group members to make a conscious choice to be witnesses for a protagonist. When both protagonist and group can hear the words of the story without triggering primitive defenses, uncontrolled regression, or unconscious abreaction, then the team leader moves on to the next principle.

OBSERVE

The second TSM principle is to observe all trauma-based roles *before* they are experienced. Having told the story, the protagonist picks people, usually TAEs, to play out the first trauma scene for observation. This gives the protagonist a chance to check for accurate portrayals of primary process reality. The trauma scene is marked, blocked out, and set in a sequence by observing the action as narrated.

The protagonist often watches the scene from the observing ego role first. Only when the protagonist can watch the whole scene without being triggered, does the team leader move on to the third principle. This gives the team a chance to provide for any additional roles needed to modify defenses to provide support for increased experiencing.

This is the time in the drama that the AL may begin to cluster group members according to their responses to the story in action. If a couple of people begin to dissociate, they could begin a "defenses cluster." When someone starts to feel like a little child, the AL gathers other people being triggered nearby. Then one team auxiliary can be assigned per cluster to help provide containment to group members.

WITNESS

The third TSM principle of conscious reexperiencing is to increase the energy of spontaneity to witness trauma-based roles from a place of feeling and connection. When this happens, the transformative role of the change agent role will emerge internally or in the group. When that happens, it is safe to move from watching the action to actively reexperiencing core trauma scenes.

Witnessing past trauma scenes often results in the protagonist spontaneously jumping in to protect his or her wounded child. The change agent role establishes that the protagonist can rescue self from the downward spiral of unprocessed trauma material. If the protagonist gets stuck in this witnessing step, it often happens that another group member begins to feel a projective identification for this needed role and spontaneously rushes in to save the wounded child. When this happens, the team leader puts the PI into action; the "good mama," or the "neighbor next door" can bring in the protective function through the healing action of group members.

The AL is responsible for structuring the increased experiencing and affective expression by the auxiliaries so that it does not overwhelm the protagonist. S/he coaches TAEs and group members alike. The AL directs spontaneous enactment of reciprocal roles that put action demands on the protagonist to rescue the wounded child in the trauma scene.

TAES act as the AL's runners. They verbally and nonverbally check with different group members to see what roles are spontaneously emerging from the energy of the group. What are they thinking? What are they feeling? What role do they feel in? Do they need a containing double? TAEs bring this clinical process information to the AL so new roles can be integrated into the action as it develops in the next principle.

REENACT

The TSM principle of reenactment provides a "walk-through" of the trauma-based scene from an active experience of one or more of the trauma-based roles. The protagonist steps into the role of victim, perpetrator, or abandoning authority and reenacts the scene slowly from this new perspective. It is a dress rehearsal for fully reexperiencing these roles in a safe and effective way.

Reenactment gives the protagonist the cognitive sequence of what will be experienced in the trauma-based role before accessing the full experiential chaos of primary process. The team leader and AL are constantly assessing the protagonist, group members, and auxiliaries for safety during reenactment. This is the last time the team will be able to set up preventive action interventions to maintain controlled regression and conscious feelings. Process assessment is completed and team members assigned for containment.

The AL directs the clusters of people in roles to increase containment and observation during reenactment scenes. The TAEs check with different group members and give the clinical and role information to the AL. The AL then decides whether to have spontaneous enactment of a role or to let the team leader know what roles are becoming available in the group through projective identification—for later action.

TAEs continue to portray the trauma-based roles as directed by the team leader. These roles are enacted without added spontaneity at this time. This is simply the first walk-through of the trauma-based role.

REEXPERIENCE

The fifth TSM principle in conscious reexperiencing is to access the state dependent learning stored in trauma bubbles for expression and full developmental repair. The roles of victim, perpetrator, and abandoning authority are safely enacted and fully experienced in the here and now of the TSM drama. For containment, most protagonists do not seek to actively experience more than one of the trauma roles at a time.

The team leader's main duty during reexperiencing is to have the proper support available for the protagonist to bring the past into the present through increases in conscious awareness. The TL constantly assesses the protagonist's ability to tolerate the increasing affect and sensorimotor representations. S/he paces the experiential work to balance cognition and affect, and adult and child ego states.

The AL monitors all other segments of the dramatic enactment that are not in the protagonist's cluster of prescriptive roles. The AL increases containment. S/he supports expression of feelings for group members when indicated. The AL works with the role clusters to keep the same cognitive/emotional balance with them that the TL keeps with the protagonist. That way, the sub-scenes that spontaneously happen during reexperiencing do not take over the protagonist's drama, but simply enhance awareness and change.

In TSM, the timing of side scenes is in fact important, but not so much from a dramatic viewpoint as the clinical perspective. The AL does not decide whether a scene will interrupt the protagonist's drama; instead, the AL asks the clinical question—does the scene need to be intervened in, and if so, using what TSM intervention module? Many times, a TSM drama is clinically stopped at different points in the sharing of a trauma bubble. Safety is of the top priority even at the cost of aesthetic production.

REPAIR

The final TSM principle in the clinical action structure of conscious reexperiencing is to enact a scene of developmental repair. Surplus reality scenes of repair are generated through the interaction of new roles and old trauma scenes. Repair scenes can focus on

- improved self-organization,
- changed childhood object relations,
- improved interpersonal relations with significant others in the present, and/or
- connections with members of the group in the here and now.

In the second half of this chapter, Tricia shares the first two scenes of a conscious reexperiencing drama she did using the Therapeutic Spiral Model. These scenes concretize the prescriptive roles, modify defenses, and develop the change agent role. They demonstrate the principles of talking, observing, and witnessing in action, which is the transition point into increased experiencing of unprocessed trauma bubbles.

TRICIA'S TSM DRAMA OF CONSCIOUS REEXPERIENCING WITH DEVELOPMENTAL REPAIR

In the real drama that this example is taken from, I am the team leader, so I use my name here. Other team members include Colette as AL, and Ann and Peter as TAEs. Wendy and Mark are auxiliaries doing training practicums. This is a typical TSM action trauma team during a *Surviving Spirits* workshop.

TSM Clinical Contract

Tricia clearly contracts for a conscious reexperiencing drama when she says, "[I] want to explore and get rid of these goddamn body memories. I know what they are. I know what happened. I just want to be free of the past now. The flashbacks are ruling my life right now and I want it back."

As team leader, I restate her goals to the team and the group:

> We are going to bring the past into the present, and see what you need to do to get free from the memories. You have built up your strengths and the group is ready to do this work with you. The team can help you consciously reexperience what your body memories are telling you. We will find new words for old experiences.

Scene 1: Enacting Prescriptive Roles for Safety

Dr. Kate/TL: Now, Tricia, I want to start the drama by you picking someone to be your containing double. (She picks Susan, another group member who knows the intervention module from previous sessions.)

Dr. Kate/TL (to Susan as she comes into the circle of safety):   You are now Tricia's containing double. You double Tricia from any role she's in, so she is not alone as she experiences the past again. You are part of her, so speak in the first person. Your job is to help her build her container with words so she doesn't get overwhelmed with feelings. You stay with her throughout the drama.

Tricia (grabs Susan's hand as she comes up to be her CD):   Oh good, I'm glad you're here. I'm really gonna need you.

Containing double: Yes, I am here and I will walk through this whole scene with you. We will do this together. You won't be alone this time.

Dr. Kate/TL: OK, Tricia, now let's pick some more help . . . is there a person in your life who can be here to walk through the past with you? Your husband? A best friend? A teacher from your childhood? Your higher power? Music? Nature? Who can help you tame these body memories?

Tricia (laughs):   Well, I am pretty self-sufficient, you know. I'm not always sure I believe in "God." I don't think I want my husband here . . . he belongs to the future, not the past. (At this moment, her body memories break through her defenses. She starts pulling at her clothes and begins to slap her thighs, looking and sounding distressed. She spontaneously says, "Oh God.")

Dr. Kate/TL (with a smile): Ah good, Tricia. Well, whether you believe in God or not, you are asking that God be here . . . what do you think? Shall we bring this "God" of yours here today? You can see if that helps or not.

Tricia (laughs): OK, OK . . . why fight it? I pick Peter (TAE) for god— that's god with a "small g"—it's not a patriarchal god, just a sense of something greater than myself . . . something beyond us humans.

Dr. Kate/TL: So, good, here's your god—with a small g. He is here on your stage today . . . tell him . . . what you need today.

Tricia: God, I would like to ask you for courage . . . and a blessing—the permission that I can do this work. (Tricia spontaneously picks up the doll she brought with her as a representation of her "inner child who doesn't have a head" and presents it to god.)

God/TAE: What is it?

Dr. Kate/TL: Role reverse and be god. God, answer that question for Tricia . . .

Tricia as god: That is my child. We are all children of god, so I give you my precious being.

TAE in protagonist role: God, is this your child?

Tricia as god: This is my child. I give her to you to cherish and take care of . . .

TAE in protagonist role: . . . to take care of and cherish. And the blessing and the courage?

Dr. Kate/TL (to Tricia in role of god): Get a scarf. I want her to have a scarf to mark your blessing. I want her to be able to remember this blessing at all times.

Tricia as god: What color is a blessing? (She chooses a pink scarf and goes to put the scarf around the doll.)

Dr. Kate/TL (to Tricia as god): No, I want the blessing around adult Tricia. She is the one doing this work today. She needs the courage, not the child of god. The child of god is beaming with light already! So, what do you say to her, god? Give your blessing to Tricia, the adult woman, so she can claim her lighted child.

Tricia as god: It's alright my child. It's safe . . . trust . . . you have a right to heal these body memories. You are my precious child.

Dr. Kate/TL: Reverse roles back to your protagonist role and receive the blessing from god now.

TAE/god: Tricia, this is my child . . . a child of god that I give to you, so that you may cherish her. This scarf is to represent courage and my blessing. Take this opportunity that you have right now. Heal the past. I will be here with you.

Tricia: I feel that . . . it's like a whole . . . great . . . big sigh of relief . . .

Colette/AL (to the group): Good, let's have a big sigh of relief. (Group members sigh out loud.) Move your arms around. Take a deep breath. Relax and connect with your own image of god in your lives.

This initial safety scene proceeds until Tricia experiences a solid sense of containment and support from people enacting the prescriptive roles that are clinically needed. In addition to god, and a CD, Tricia picks people for a body double, and a lion of courage. She says the group is her interpersonal support.

Looking at the AL, for a quick assessment of the rest of the group, and getting a nod, I clinically decide we can end Scene 1. The prescriptive roles are available. Tricia is connected to her body, mind, emotions, and spirit as an adult woman. She is supported by the group. As team leader, I direct the clinical focus from restoration and containment to observation of a trauma-based scene as Scene 2 begins.

Scene 2: Modifying Defenses and Finding the Change Agent

Dr. Kate/TL: OK, we are ready to move into Scene 2. Let's begin to bring the past into the present here in our circle of safety. What scene, fragments, sounds, etc., do you want to experience here? You have your CD and other roles here to help you. What do you choose to explore?

Tricia (with her CD and BD standing right next to her, yet sounding like a child): I was told . . . about . . . me . . . when I was little . . . by my sister . . . my older sister. We were sent to church by our parents; they didn't go, but we were sent. And on our way home from church on Sundays, my sister told me that she would take me to the outside edge of town . . . oh, I don't know how old I was . . . and say, "Go that way and don't ever come back." I don't remember that. (She looks sad and tearful and a bit agitated.)

And I was told that I used to wet my pants and hang the underpants on the bushes to dry. (She looks nervous and scared and has increasing unconscious body movements).

And I was told that, it was in Nova Scotia, and it was cold, and it was wintertime . . . there was a family next door that had a little baby . . . a baby they would put out in the baby carriage in the daytime. I was told that I would go and undress the baby and leave the baby in the cold.

As Tricia reports this third incident, body memories overwhelm her and she starts to regress. Her voice tone shifts to one of panic and anxiety. She pulls at her clothes, twisting and turning around, looking ashamed. Her face looks like a little girl.

The TL touches the arms of the prescriptive roles to interrupt the uncontrolled regression.

CD: It's OK for me to talk about these things I was told about me as a kid. I am an adult now. I can make sense of the past. I can pay attention to my body memories in a new way.

Body double: I can feel my feet on the ground. My breathing is going in and out. I can feel my life force in my breath. I can walk around my space.

Dr. Kate/TL (checking for the contract and informed consent):   Tricia, here is a good place to take a breath. Do you want to continue?

Tricia (shifts back to her adult ego state stabilizing the protagonist role):   OK, yes, I *can* take a deep breath. I am an adult now. But this is just what I meant. Here I am just talking about what I was told about my past . . . and I feel like a little girl with my body jumping all over the place! This is *exactly* what I want to stop.

Dr. Kate/TL: Shall we explore this scene more in action then? It certainly did trigger your body memories, so there must be some connection between them.

Tricia cognitively contracts to explore this childhood scene when she was 5 years old and undressed the baby of the neighbor (a Colonel). We will use the principles of conscious reexperiencing for developmental repair. The remainder of Scene 2 takes us through the principles of talk, observe, and witness; all the steps that need to be completed prior to actively reexperiencing the trauma roles directly.

Tricia: Yes, I can do that with the help of my CD . . . my god . . . the group. OK, let's do it. What do we do next?

Talk

Dr. Kate/TL: Let's go to that scene with the Colonel's baby. How old are you?

Tricia: I don't know.

Dr. Kate/TL: You might know . . . you may not know consciously in your mind . . . in your intellect . . . but what about your intuition and the felt body sense of your experience?

Tricia: Five or six?

Dr. Kate/TL: Your heart knows?

Tricia (smiles):   Right!

Dr. Kate/TL: Yeah, your heart knows. You have a great heart, good intuition . . . your heart knows 5 or 6. That's what we have to trust here—your body knowing, your feelings, your primary process. We're not looking for answers here (points to head), but here (heart) and here (gut).

We'll get back to your head and its meanings later. Right now we are just trying out some ideas you have so you can decide for yourself what is real. Let's set up that scene.

Tricia: OK.

Dr. Kate/TL: OK, so what I'd like you to do is to pick Ann or Wendy (TAEs) to be the baby in the crib.

Tricia: Ann . . . she looks so childlike.

Dr. Kate/TL: So tell us what we are going to see. Ann will be the Colonel's baby. You will pick someone to be your 5-year-old self. What will we see?

Tricia: I don't know why, but I want to see myself undressing the Colonel's baby and leaving it out in the cold like my sister always said I did. I want to see how that is connected to these damn body memories.

Dr. Kate/TL: OK, let's set up the crib. Let's build the crib somehow . . . you can use scarves, chairs, pillows . . . it's not a crib, right, it's a baby carriage?

Tricia: It's a baby carriage . . . like those old prams they have in England. They didn't have purple for babies in those days . . . white. She puts several chairs together and drapes them with white scarves. (Without thought, Tricia picks up her doll and throws her into the crib she has created.)

Dr. Kate/TL: . . . you put the child of god in the pram, too?

Tricia: Yes, I guess I did. Well, she belongs there it seems. (At this moment Tricia compulsively bursts away from the pram and begins shaking her arm up and down, moaning in pain.)

Dr. Kate/TL: What just happened, Tricia?

Tricia (with BD and CD next to her, she starts to ego state shift and her voice becomes very hostile): Oh, that's just the Colonel's baby, she's always out there in the cold crying . . . I don't care about her.

Dr. Kate/TL: Well, what is happening with your arm?

Tricia (with prescriptive roles by her side): Oh, my arm hurts . . . my arm hurts . . .

Tricia then rushes back in toward the pram scene and pulls the doll out of Ann's arms. There is compulsive action here as she moves toward the pram with aggression, hostility, and a change in her voice. She is experientially organizing around alternating victim and perpetrator ego states in the here and now.

Tricia (in 5-year-old ego state): Give me that doll. That's not your doll. It's mine. (She tosses the doll on the floor.)

CD: Whoa, what just happened here? All of a sudden I felt like I was a little girl again, back here with the Colonel's baby. Now, I can also feel that I am an adult today, here in this group.

BD: I can look around at the group members here. I can take a deep breath and feel my energy shift from that child place. I can feel my adult arms and legs.

Tricia (looking a bit stunned and slowly moving her eyes to look at each group member): OK, yes . . . I'm here now. I'm not sure what just happened.

Tricia has shown some uncontrolled regression and compulsive acting out as she talked about this trauma scene. She has however, compensated quickly, with the help of her prescriptive roles. As team leader, I decide to continue to increase active experiencing of roles of observation—to increase cognitive awareness and narrative labeling—before progressing further down the spiral into unconscious memories.

Observe

Dr. Kate/TL: Role reverse into your observing ego role. Stand by your OE cards and let's observe this scene. Bring your containing and body doubles with you so you can stay in your adult state. Where do you want god and your courageous lion to be?

Tricia as OE (she sits down in a chair):   I want god right behind me with his hand on my shoulder. The lion, he can lie down in front of me and keep an eye on things.

Dr. Kate/TL to team: Ann, get out of the crib. Put the doll, the child of god, back in the crib. Take the role of 5-year-old Tricia and walk through what she just showed us happened. Use a tinge of the hostile voice tone and the compulsive actions you observed. Just walk it through, so we can check for accuracy and containment.

Colette/AL assesses the level of containment in other group members during this initial enactment of a trauma-based scene. She asks several people, who have begun to dissociate in the face of the hostility and compulsive energy, to sit together in a cluster. She asks Mark to take on the role of CD for people trying to stay present right now.

Mark makes CD statements for them as a group: It's OK. I can watch this scene. It may remind me of something in my own life, but I can stay present . . . and watch this with Tricia. It is her story and I can see similarities and differences with mine. I am in the present, here and now in this TSM group.

Dr. Kate/TL: Tricia, stop here for a moment. Come stand beside me and let's watch what just happened. Ann, you become Tricia as the 5-year-old. Start with your arm hurting with body memories. Show us the scene where she regresses and goes in and grabs the doll and then tosses her aside. Tricia, what do you notice here from this place of observation?

Tricia/OE: There is aggression . . . that's all I was ever used to . . .

Dr. Kate/TL: So, you were doing to the baby what was done to you?

Tricia/OE: Yeah, that's all I ever knew . . . violence, hitting, sexual abuse. No, that's not true. I also remember wonderful parties. Fancy dinners. Daddy's powerful friends. It was all very confusing.

Witness

Dr. Kate/TL: OK, so right now, let's watch this scene again and sort out the confusion. We can witness what happened to you as a child here in the present with the group and see what is important, OK? (I direct Ann to start the scene and increase her affect and actions to put action demands on Tricia for the change agent role.)

Ann as hostile, out-of-control 5-year-old: I don't care about that baby. I have to throw her out of the pram. She doesn't belong there. I'm gonna pick her up and tell her never to come back here again! (When Ann as 5-year-old Tricia picks up the child of god and is going to throw it on the floor, god steps in and loudly interrupts the action.)

God/TAE to 5-year-old: Stop. That is my child of god. Do not treat her like that. Tricia, (he turns to adult/protagonist Tricia in the OE role) what is happening here?

Dr. Kate/TL: Hold the action here. Now Tricia, as an adult, you can answer that question of god's. You can see from this adult witness role what your 5-year-old child role did. Tell god what you see and what you need from him for yourself or your child.

Tricia/OE: Oh . . . I see that I tossed the child of god out of the pram. I didn't care. I sounded just like my father . . . that was his voice filled with hatred. He was both so wonderful and so horrid. But I remember that hatred in his voice. It was like he was speaking through me. Yuck!

CD: I can see these connections and stay in the present. I can connect the body memory in my arm to my father's hatred, and see my wanting to hurt the Colonel's baby in a new way. Today, I'm not hurting any-one . . . not myself, not others. I am just looking at my life.

Tricia/OE to god: It is good you stopped the child. She doesn't know any different. Bring her to you and tell her she's OK.

Dr. Kate/TL: Tricia, role reverse into your 5-year-old wounded child role. Now, god, say that to little Tricia again so she can hear and understand you. Like big Tricia said, bring her to you and tell her she's OK.

God/TAE: Come here, Tricia. You are a precious child of god. I don't want you to be hurt. I don't want you to hurt others. Come here and let me hold your hand.

Five-year-old Tricia (looks up at god with tears in her eyes):   I really don't want to hurt the Colonel's baby. I don't want to hurt anyone. Am I OK?

God/TAE: Yes, I know you don't want to hurt anyone. Come here, take my hand. (She tentatively gets up and walks over to god and offers her hand, still looking small.) You are precious. No one should ever hurt you. Today I am here to help protect you. You are OK. You are OK with me. (The change agent role has emerged.)

Five-year-old Tricia: Thank you. Thank you. I wasn't always sure you existed, but today I think maybe you do. (She cries for a bit while god holds her hand, pats it, and says soothing words.)

Dr. Kate/TL: Reverse back now into your protagonist role. Step out of the wounded child and listen to this final sentence between little Tricia and god.

In this scene, Peter's spontaneous action as god develops the transformative role of the change agent. When the protagonist was unable to rescue herself, the TAE stepped in to break the trauma pattern of self-abandonment. Comfort was given and appropriate authority taken by god. With the change agent present, the team knows we can now make the transition into experiencing trauma-based roles directly. Tricia has shown that even when triggered, she can draw on her prescriptive roles and the TL's directions for structure.

CONCLUSIONS

Chapter 7 first detailed the 5th clinical action structure in the TSM: the six principles of conscious reexperiencing. Each action step was demonstrated by clients to show the clinical decision making points built in for safety and controlled regression.

Then, this chapter presented the first three steps in conscious reexperiencing for developmental repair in TSM: talk, observe, and witness.

Tricia shared the first two scenes in a drama about accessing, expressing, and labeling body memories. She was able to utilize her prescriptive roles and to modify her use of identification with the aggressor as a defense. She is now ready to increase her own active experiencing of trauma-based roles with the support of the group and the term.

CHAPTER EIGHT

Conscious Reexperiencing of the Victim Role: Scenes 3–6

CHAPTER OVERVIEW

This chapter continues to follow Tricia's story of healing, using the clinical action structures of the Therapeutic Spiral Model. It presents the last three principles of conscious reexperiencing, that address enactment of trauma-based roles: reenact, reexperience, and repair.

TRICIA'S TSM DRAMA OF CONSCIOUS REEXPERIENCING OF THE VICTIM ROLE

As Tricia takes the role of the Colonel's baby, she accesses unprocessed information about her own childhood sexual abuse. The principles of conscious reexperiencing are then repeated with this second trauma scene in Tricia's life. She experiences a controlled regression to her own 3-year-old wounded child. She expresses long dissociated feelings and achieves developmental repair. We celebrate integration of her sleeping-awakening child, who has become fully awake and aware of her intelligence and beauty!

Prior to this scene, Tricia concretized her prescriptive roles (Scene 1). When she slipped into compulsive reenactment and ego state changes, she found the transformative role of a change agent in her "god." She observed and witnessed the scene she is now ready to enact (Scene 2). She is willing to take the victim role in her TSM drama for conscious reexperiencing with developmental repair. She hopes to make sense of the past and stop the flashbacks and body memories in the present.

SCENE THREE: CONSCIOUS REEXPERIENCING OF VICTIM ROLE—THE COLONEL'S BABY

Reenact

Dr. Kate/TL: OK, what I want you to do is role reverse with Colonel Jones's baby, keeping your CD and BD with you so you're not going back into the past alone. God and the lion of courage are here if you need them. Let's bring the scene from the past into the present to learn what you need to know. Role reverse with Colonel Jones' baby. Beside you in this pram is this child of god.

Dr. Kate/TL (assigns Wendy [AE] to the new role): I want you to come over here . . . and I want you to be the child of god that's also in this crib. But you don't have a face for Tricia, so you're a child of god—without a face. Tricia, you take the role of the Colonel's baby in the pram.

Ann is role reversed into the role of the 5-year-old Tricia, and I put an empty chair in to hold the protagonist/client role for Tricia to reverse back to if needed to increase cognitive functioning.

Dr. Kate/TL to team: OK, set the drama into action with Tricia here in the role of the Colonel's baby. The child of god is next to her. Ann is playing Tricia at 5 years old. Walk it through so she can feel what happens without getting overwhelmed.

Ann/5 year old: My daddy told me not to do that, but I have to . . . I have to go . . . I'm going to do it . . . here's that baby . . . (compulsive energy, hostile tone alternating with needy child voice).

Dr. Kate/TL (to Tricia as she begins to take the role of the Colonel's baby): Hear the energy coming toward you. You're a little baby without words to know what is happening. Five-year-old Tricia is coming toward you . . .

As team leader, I direct the prescriptive doubles to increase their narrative labeling at this point in the drama. This helps Tricia to maintain the cognitive ability to label what is happening as each and every trauma bubble is accessed and slowly opened.

CD: I can stay present both to my experience here in this role as the Colonel's baby . . . and I can see what little Tricia is about as well. I am scared and I can still look at what I am learning today. Both adult and child roles are present.

BD: I can feel my body against the chair here. I am not a few months old in a pram. I am in a TSM drama using props to help me make sense of these body memories. I am OK.

Dr. Kate/TL: OK, let's continue to experience a bit more of what the role of the baby is here in your drama. See how it is connected to your body memories, the ones you want to stop. (I direct Ann to increase her action demands for active experiencing and we move to the next principle of conscious reexperiencing.)

Reexperience

TAE/5-year-old: I take this baby's clothes off . . . take this off . . . get that doll.

Tricia/Colonel Jones's baby: Don't touch me. Don't touch me. Nooooooo! (Starts to cry.)

Body double: I can feel both the sense of this baby body and remember my adult body. I can keep my eyes open and see what is happening today.

Ann/5-year-old Tricia: I just want to touch the baby . . . I just want to touch the baby . . . (repeating words Tricia compulsively said in the role of her 5-year-old child.)

As TL, I have assessed that Tricia has the ego strength and the necessary supporting auxiliary egos to continue the exploration. The decision here is to structure controlled regression in the service of the ego.

Dr. Kate/TL: Hold the action. Baby, who is this person? Who are you so scared of?

Tricia with CD/BD in role of baby (She begins to cry and screams):   No, NO . . . NO . . . Don't touch me!

I see Tricia shifting states of consciousness, experiencing the bridge between her regressed and dissociated child state and an adult self that is able to reflect on what is happening and find words to express it. The adult self opens her eyes with surprise and reports quite clearly as follows:

Tricia/baby role (with surprise and sadness): Oh, my father . . . my father . . . it's my father!

Dr. Kate/TL: It's your father?

Tricia (in a co-conscious state of baby and adult roles, with congruent affect of horror and sadness): Yes . . . and I can feel him against my back. Against my rectum . . . against my back! Ohhhhhhh, God! (Dr. Kate/TL directs god/TAE to repeat his protective change agent role here.)

God/TAE: Tricia, Tricia, I am here with you. See me. I will not let it happen to you again. Tell me, how old are you?

Tricia: I don't know.

Dr. Kate/TL: Are you a baby? Are you older?

Tricia in a co-conscious state: No, I'm maybe 3 . . . I don't know . . . why would he want to do that? I don't know . . .

God/TAE: You are 3 years old and you are my precious child of god. You are OK. I'll be here with you.

Dr. Kate/TL: Hold this scene. We have the choice to stop here. You found out how the scene with the Colonel's baby related to your arm hurting. Now we see that it is also connected to your own sexual abuse. Do you want to go to the next trauma bubble or not?

Tricia responds that she does want to proceed, knowing we will use the principles of conscious reexperiencing to now explore this core trauma scene in her own life.

SCENE FOUR: NARRATIVE LABELING AND WITNESSING OF CORE VICTIM ROLE

Dr. Kate/TL: OK, let's start this next scene from outside the 3-year-old role. Role reverse into your OE again. (I direct Tricia away from the space that is marked for the pram and to the chair that has held the protagonist/client role. It is still next to her OE cards that are on the wall.)

Dr. Kate/TL to Tricia: We are going to put Wendy (TAE) in as your wounded 3-year-old child. She's going to play that role so you don't have to do it. Sit here with me, with the support of your containing and body doubles. Let's have god and your courageous lion nearby as well.

Wendy's going to be that part that you're remembering . . . the 3-year-old; so you don't have to, OK? You just remembered something? What did you remember? Let's watch from the safety of distance. Take the role of your observing ego again.

Talk

Tricia/OE role: Well, I just remember it starting, but I don't remember anything other than that.

Dr. Kate/TL: So, you remember it starting . . . your father against your back? Your rectum?

Tricia/OE role (voices shifts again, becomes hostile and seems to come from the internalization of her father):   Yeah, I liked it . . . (goes flat; no voice tone or affect at all), but when it comes to the part when he actually . . . does it, there isn't anything there.

(In her adult voice) What I think we will see is him sexually abusing me. Hurting me. Degrading me. Maybe I really don't want to see this.

Dr. Kate/TL: Of course, we can stop here if you want.

Tricia/OE role: Let's keep going.

Observe

Dr. Kate/TL: We're just going to take this one step at a time . . . OK? I want to remind you where we are in the drama: in the role of the Colonel's baby, you said, and I'm just checking this out . . . what you said is that . . . he was behind you at your rectum and when I asked you how old you were you said 3 . . . and then you spontaneously regressed and went to another scene and your body went wild (pause) and you said it was your father sexually abusing you? (Tricia nods and grabs her CD's hand.) So let's just watch that scene and see what it means to you today, how it connects with your body memories.

Witness

Dr. Kate/TL: What I want is—Ann, you are here as Tricia's 3-year-old self who has a face, and you, Wendy, are in here as the baby who doesn't have a face yet. Now Tricia, we need to ask someone to play Dad. You can ask group members and they may say no. Mark is available if he fits for you.

Tricia: Mark will do just fine.

Mark takes the role of the father. He moves up behind 3-year-old Tricia who is played by both Ann and Wendy (all team members). They are concretizing a split in self organization—between the faceless baby (victim role) and the child of god (sleeping-awakening child).

Mark/Dad/TAE: She likes it. Yes, she does . . .

Tricia/OE role: No, I don't want it!

Dad/TAE (repeating words Tricia said):   Yes, she does; I've been telling her over and over how she likes it.

Wendy/wounded-headless child: No, no (rocks nonverbally and begins to wail).

Dad/TAE: She likes it and I'm going to show her what it's really like.

Wendy/wounded-headless child: No, no . . . NOOOOOOOOOOOOOOOO! Oh God, help me!

God/TAE: Stop it—Father! You cannot do this to your daughter! It is not right! Stop, right now. I said STOP!

Dr. Kate/TL: OK, Tricia, hold the action scene here.

Tricia/OE (spontaneously starts to cry as she is supported by her CD and other prescriptive roles):   Oh that was so awful . . . I could feel exactly how he was . . . it's like he still lives inside me . . . I feel so awful.

Dr. Kate/TL: Auxiliaries, support her and tell her she's OK. Give Tricia the messages from your prescriptive role.

As Tricia completes the principle of witnessing her trauma scene, I assess that we are not ready to move to further conscious reexperiencing of her victim role yet. Instead, I direct Tricia to experience an action structure for developmental repair first.

Repair

CD: It's OK, I am not my father. I can feel myself as I am now as an adult who survived this abuse. I am hurting. I can feel the hurt. I am not hateful and cruel. I am hurting. It is OK to cry even though I am scared. We are together in this now.

Unconditional Love (a role that developed spontaneously by a group member from the action): Tricia, no matter what happened to you, I still love you . . . you are worthy of love. It is good to get this out in the open . . . you're OK. Just take some deep breaths and breathe in my safe warm love.

This scene of developmental repair occurs until Tricia is well resourced. She is in contact with her prescriptive and transformative roles, and ready to continue down the therapeutic spiral again. The role of unconditional love has been added to her role atom now.

Because the protagonist has demonstrated that she can stay present to both the victim and perpetrator roles, I ask her which trauma role she needs to experience for her healing today. Tricia spontaneously picks up her doll and makes the decision to reexperience her trauma scene from the wounded-headless child role, which is the one she knows the least. This is the true victim representation of core traumatic experience, and I assess that she is ready to go to the deepest levels of the spiral for full developmental repair.

Scene Five: Conscious Reexperiencing of Core Victim Role—Tricia's 3-Year-Old Child

Dr. Kate/TL: So, what are we going to create here? What scene will make a difference in your life?

Tricia in protagonist role: . . . Rosalie . . . (she picks up her doll once again).

Dr. Kate/TL: Rosalie?

Tricia: Yes, Rosalie's my name. Patricia Rose is my given name. Rosalie was my nickname until I was 12. Then I decided to call myself Tricia.

Dr. Kate/TL: OK, so this (points to the doll) is Rosalie?

Tricia: Yes, this Rosalie.

Dr. Kate/TL: Uh-huh . . . but without the face? Is this Rosalie with or without a face?

Tricia (She is again triggered into uncontrolled regression and doubles over in pain, holding her stomach. She has unconsciously walked from the observing space to the place on stage marked for her bedroom as a 3-year-old child. She cries.):   . . . oh, my vagina hurts . . .

Dr. Kate/TL: OK, your vagina is hurting. OK, where can we sit so that we can safely experience this?

As TL I assess that Tricia can in fact go with the regression that has been triggered after being resourced by her scene of developmental repair. Her drama is, after all, about her body memories. She has the support of her auxiliaries and I direct the team to directly proceed with the principle of conscious reexperiencing.

Reexperience

CD: I can sit down right here. My vagina does hurt. I feel awful, like that little kid again. This time I can also keep my adult self around. I know I will get through this. This is what I came to do, to sort out what triggers these body memories so I can make them stop.

Courageous lion: Don't anyone start messing with Tricia here. She is in pain. She is hurting. And I will protect her and destroy anyone who tries to come near her. ROAR!

Body double: I can hear the roar of the lion. I can take a deep breath and remember I am in a TSM group right now. I am not back in the past. Let me look around and connect with the eyes of one of my friends here today. I can choose to bring the past into the present.

Tricia (in a controlled regression. She is crying and yelling, twisting on the floor, holding herself, in tears):   I want my vagina! I want it . . . I want it . . . I want it . . . I want it for me—not for him!

Dr. Kate/TL: Say that again.

Tricia (with support of her prescriptive roles):   I want my vagina for me. I don't want him to have it . . . it's mine, it's mine . . .

Dr. Kate/TL: How old are you now?

Tricia (alternating child and adult roles):   I don't know how old I am. It's mine, it's mine, it's not yours . . . I'm just a little girl!

Tricia consciously abreacts in her 3-year-old role until she fully releases dissociated feelings of terror, horror, rage, and despair from her body. She calms down naturally as her energy ebbs. With her prescriptive and transformative roles on hand, she orients to the here and now fully. She is in the circle of safety, doing a conscious reexperiencing drama using the Therapeutic Spiral Model. There is no rush here. Tricia gently receives support and containment from the people playing her prescriptive and transformative roles.

Repair

God/TAE: I am here with you. You can feel your childhood feelings and know you're not alone.

Lion: I'll devour anyone who ever tries to hurt you again.

Body double: I can feel my body. It is *my* body. All of it is my body. No one else can have it. No one can touch me without my permission, not ever again! I feel my adult body. I can feel my fingers and toes. I can move them. I can feel the muscles in my arms. I am a strong woman.

Tricia: Yes, I can experience the difference between then and now. It is my body. It is my vagina. Maybe that is what my body memories were trying to tell me . . . this is my body. No one else can have it but me.

Having now experienced the meaning of her body memories with their attendant fears and rages, the repair scene needs to be further anchored in. I direct Tricia back to the principle of witnessing to increase narrative labeling of her healing experience. Together we look at the aftermath of her controlled regression on self-organization. We put words to what we see.

Witness

Dr. Kate/TL: Let's watch the controlled regression from your adult role to your wounded child role. You can see what happened with your body memories and feelings. You can put new words on your experience of being sexually abused by your father. That way, you don't have to keep going through uncontrolled regression, obsessive thinking, and unconscious feelings over and over again.

  Look at this scene now. During the body memories you just experienced, Ann/the child of god role spontaneously split off from the trauma scene. She got scared and ran off, but she is still here. She is watching and waiting from a safe place outside the circle of experiencing. She is looking for you.

Wendy, your headless wounded child is still covered up by the defenses. She is dissociated and unconnected to self or others. She has given up all hope.

This time, however, we will see that you and god stopped the abuse. You claimed back your body. Let's use this power you found to bring all of your parts together, OK?

Tricia: Yes, I still want to find my face.

Thus, we begin the final scene of developmental repair.

SCENE SIX: DEVELOPMENTAL REPAIR

Repair in Self-Organization

Tricia in protagonist role (with deep longing in her voice):   Oh, I want a face so bad . . .

(Ann comes down from the balcony where she has stayed while the trauma scene was enacted—split off but aware. She enacts the projective identification of the child of god/the TSM awakening child role.)

Ann: I'm here, you found me . . .

Tricia: I haven't had a head . . .

Ann/child of god (comes down to the bottom step, picks up the doll, and holds her out to adult Tricia):   You found me.

Tricia: I haven't had a head, it's been all disconnected.

Ann/child of god: Here I am . . . (As director, I indicate for her to stay at the foot of the stairs, so Tricia will have to take the action of integration herself).

Tricia (turns and looks at her child of god):   Where do I go?

Ann/child of god (she motions toward the stage where the wounded-headless child self is still covered up on the floor):   . . . right here . . .

Dr. Kate/TL: First, you have to open up the blankness . . . first . . . there's the blankness . . .

(Tricia slowly takes the scarves off the faceless child.)

Dr. Kate/TL (directs Ann/child of God to concretize the integration of the split self-representations):   Put your face right down next to her, next to the wounded child Wendy is playing.

Wendy/wounded-headless child: I was so scared . . .

Dr. Kate/TL (to Tricia, motioning to the faces):   I want you to see the horror and terror on this face, the wounded child (pause, look at Wendy) and the innocence on this face, your awakening child (pause, look at Ann), and blend them. This is how you give Rosalie back her face. Yes, take this one (the child of god) and put it on there (wounded child), so you can have your face back.

Ann/child of god (to Tricia):   Only you can do it.

Tricia (to child of god with a surprised smile and a sigh of relief): You're beautiful!

Dr. Kate/TL: Yes, alright, that's you—you're talking to your 3-year-old self now.

Ann/child of god: Oh, I'm so glad you found me!

There is a true moment of healing and developmental repair as Tricia touches the face of her child of god, and Ann, the auxiliary, cries through her shining face at the beauty of the spontaneous acceptance.

Dr. Kate/TL (to Tricia):   Just look at the beauty of that 3-year-old child . . . your face. Now, I want you to role reverse and come down here (points to the floor as Ann gets up to role reverse). I want you to come over here and get your face given back. This is Rosalie's new heritage.

I role reverse Tricia into the child of god role. She experiences this moment of recognition and acceptance. The split is healing from both sides of the primary process representations—the adult and the child states. A new personal narrative is created.

Ann as protagonist (reaching out and touching Tricia's face):   Rosalie? (pause) Rosalie? Rosalie . . . come over here, I need you. (Ann pulls Tricia's head very close to the faceless child who has been uncovered.) Can I find you? Are you here? Can I find you?

Tricia as Rosalie/child of god: Mhm mhm.

Ann as protagonist: Can I turn this over? (Tricia's doll—the blank side to the face side)

Tricia as Rosalie/child of god (rolls onto her back. Clapping, with a huge smile lighting her face):   I have a head! I have a head! I have a head! I just got a head! (Everybody is clapping.)

Dr. Kate/TL: Alright! Feel that head. (Then to Ann still in protagonist role) Come to Rosalie's face. Tell her how beautiful she is.

Ann as protagonist: You're beautiful . . . you're beautiful!

Tricia experiences action insight and we can see healing occur right before our eyes. There is spontaneity and connection throughout the group. A collective sense of awe fills the room. Group members turn to each other with love and compassion in their eyes.

Tricia as Rosalie/child of god (sitting up, clapping and smiling):   Oh, I got a head . . . I got a head . . . I got a head . . . a head . . . a head on my body!

Ann as protagonist (touching Tricia/Rosalie's hair and face with wonder):   Oh yes, a whole head . . .

Tricia as Rosalie/child of god: Yes, a whole head. I don't have a slit neck anymore . . . a whole body!

Ann as protagonist: Yes, yes, ears . . . eyes . . . nose . . . chin . . . Is there hair back here too?

Dr. Kate/TL: Reverse roles. Ann, you become the awakening child. Tricia, you come back to the protagonist role.

Tricia/Rosalie/protagonist: I think I can make the journey now. I think . . . I can take all parts of me with me. They're not quite together . . . I have a little scoop of a face and it's trying to get on the body and it's trying to skip along.

Dr. Kate/TL: Well, we have one more way we can help you get your face anchored into the present. Let's face the group and I want anyone who can come up and welcome your new face to do so. This will help you keep your face on your body. (A group member approaches with a mirror.)

Dr. Kate/TL: Look here, you've got a gift . . . ?

Andrea (who played the body double):   Everybody else sees your real face, your changed face . . . now it's your turn to see your changed face (holds a mirror so Tricia can see).

Tricia (surprised, clapping, smiling, with a few tears): Oh, it does look pretty good! (Everybody claps.)

Tricia (touches both faces, her wounded child and her child of god): Yes, you are both part of me. I see my beauty in Rosalie. I was such a lovely child. And I see my pain in the wounded child. But together they make up me. And I see I have a head now! I am OK.

Dr. Kate/TL: Great, this is a good place to stop. Let's sit down and have some sharing.

Sharing

Colette/AL: I found myself watching you so closely when you gathered your lion, your god, and your doubles around you for protection. I find that the more I do the TSM work, the more I am aware of my "protectors." Thank you for reminding me to draw on them in my times of need.

Andrea/BD: When I saw your body go crazy with pain, I was horrified at first. I know that is what my body wants to do, but I keep it under such control with my anorexia, it cannot. I could see the pain and terror pouring out of your body. And there you were screaming, "I want my body. It is mine." That gave me so much courage. I think I might be able to do a scene where I claim my body back from the boys who raped me. Thank you so much for showing me the way.

Jim: I really identified with how your higher power saved you. Most of the time you didn't even notice he was there . . . but each time when the abuse was gonna happen again, that's who stepped in. It was god that stopped the cycle of violence in your life and it's God that has stopped it in mine.

I saw your innocent child and I knew—I have one of them too. I could always see God in the guys at the house. Them, I can see God shining right through them. But it's always been hard for me to see myself that way. But I saw how you brought that faceless child and the child of light together. That worked for me. Thanks.

Ann/TAE: I want to thank you for the privilege of being your child of god. I was truly awakened in that role. It was great to be seen, brought alive, and fully accepted. I was really touched by that experience today.

As a mother of two young girls, I give a lot of unconditional love to them. And sometimes as a Mom, I need a little refill myself. Today, I feel like I was blessed and loved. Thank you.

Peter/TAE: I deeply appreciate playing your god. I am not always sure what I think or experience about god in my own life. I do believe in something that guides me. I just don't know what to call it, I guess. Anyway, in that role, I knew that the only important thing was to stop violence from repeating itself whenever I could. That was my job.

I feel that way about this TSM work we do. This work makes a difference for people. We do help stop cycles of violence. That matters to me. When I discovered psychodrama, through my cousin, it changed my life. I am always happy to be part of a TSM drama when it changes someone else's life. Thank you. It was a renewal of faith and love for me today.

Vladamir: Yes, that is part of what I got out of your drama today, Tricia. It renewed for me my belief that healing can actually happen. Some days at the refugee center, I think I cannot go on. There is too much trauma. Too much loss. Too much sadness. I think of my family and what I have lost. I feel like I cannot go on anymore. It is too much.

Being with you in your drama today as you bravely faced your past, your trauma bubbles . . . it has given me courage.

The rest of the team members and group participants share their strength, hope, and experience from the TSM drama of conscious reexperiencing with developmental repair. More tears are shared. Hugs are exchanged. A tangible sense of hope fills the group.

CONCLUSIONS

This chapter completes Tricia's TSM drama of conscious reexperiencing with developmental repair. It is a good example of how the clinical action structures of TSM guide experiential therapy with trauma survivors diagnosed with PTSD. Tricia's drama of conscious reexperiencing demonstrated the process of spiraling in and out of trauma material to create new meanings in the present. The TSIRA guided implementation of prescriptive, trauma-based, and transformative roles as the clinical map for action methods with PTSD. Even the role of victim was concretized, experienced, and changed. Dissociated feelings were released. The developmental repair of surplus reality transformed the past with life-affirming images for the future.

CHAPTER NINE

Processing Tricia's Drama: Advanced Action Intervention Modules in Scenes 1 and 2

CHAPTER OVERVIEW

Chapters 7 and 8 brought Tricia's drama of conscious experiencing with developmental repair alive for the readers. This chapter processes Scenes 1 and 2 in Tricia's drama demonstrating the final clinical action structure in TSM: the advanced action intervention modules.

Fourteen separate interventions have been developed in TSM to guide practice following the clinical map of the trauma survivor's intrapsychic role atom. In some cases interventions are as simple as enacting a role, for example, the observing ego role or the courageous lion in Tricia's drama. For others, there is a step-by-step clinical structure that guides the practitioner using TSM. In several cases, the intervention modules have been operationalized and tested.

Presented here are six of the TSM intervention modules that were used in Scenes 1 and 2. The first three developed the following prescriptive roles in Tricia's drama:

- the body double,
- the containing double, and
- the keeper of defenses.

These TSM prescriptive interventions provided containment of body memories, emotional flashbacks, and primitive defenses for Tricia. This chapter also processes how the drama established the following transformative roles:

- the sleeping-awakening child,
- the change agent, and
- the manager of healthy functioning.

Together with the restorative roles, the observing ego, and the client role, these advanced TSM intervention modules provided containment, resiliency, and adaptive functioning prior to increased experiencing of trauma-based roles in Tricia's drama.

PROCESSING THE DRAMA

In classical psychodrama there are a number of ways to "process a drama." The standard format is to follow the director's decision making from start to finish, that is through warm-up, action, and sharing (Hollander, 1969). Sometimes, a drama is sociometrically processed (Hale, 1985), noting who played each role and what their connection was to the protagonist. Social atoms and cultural atoms can both be used as assessment tools after a psychodrama as well as before (Moreno, 1977).

In the Therapeutic Spiral Model, team leaders most often process dramas using the trauma survivor's intrapsychic role atom. As the clinical map that guides all TSM intervention modules, the TSIRA is an excellent template for accessing change before, during, and after a drama. To have a full understanding of the use of TSM interventions, this chapter details a director's soliloquy, technique description, and comments on the team roles for each intervention used in Tricia's drama.

SCENE 1: ENACTING PRESCRIPTIVE ROLES FOR SAFETY

Please refer to chapter 7 for the description and dialogue of Scenes 1 and 2 in Tricia's drama. Scene 1 demonstrates the emergence of the prescriptive and transformative roles needed to face the unconscious trauma material held in body memories.

DIRECTOR'S SOLILOQUY

As Tricia and I walk and talk in the circle of safety, we set up a contract for conscious reexperiencing with developmental repair. I repeat it out loud to make sure that everyone hears what she will work on. My words let the team know that the drama will spiral into the past, to her childhood, for the purpose of finding new endings to old memories. The team is aware of the need for containment and pacing given the depth of the clinical contract.

As team leader in Scene 1, my entire focus is on enacting Tricia's prescriptive roles as they are needed to face her story of trauma. This is one of the main differences from classical psychodrama. During this first scene I do not follow the protagonist's lead as s/he talks about a trauma. I am not thinking about how to put the trauma scene into action. Instead, in TSM, the director/team leader listens to the story the protagonist wants to put into action, and clinically decides what prescriptive roles need to be enacted so that trauma scenes can happen safely. Considerations of diagnosis, treatment planning, and timing are also integrated into clinical directing in TSM.

Tricia had been diagnosed with PTSD when she first sought treatment. At the time of her drama, she had already internalized most of the prescriptive roles, at least to some degree. I knew she was safe to open some trauma bubbles. I also knew that she highly valued her mind and her ability to make sense of things. That let me know I would definitely need a containing double for her to increase cognitive processing throughout her drama. She was working on body memories—she'd need a body double. I prescribed both prescriptive doubles early in the drama. The other prescriptive roles? I would wait and see what she spontaneously produced and put them into action at that time.

In fact, Tricia was able to spontaneously produce two roles in Scene 1: her image of God (god; a restorative role of transpersonal strength), and a doll to represent herself as a precious child of god (the transformative role of the sleeping-awakening child). This level of spontaneity and creativity showed that her prescriptive roles were well integrated and able to be used in the face of trauma.

As team leader, I made sure I did not get seduced into trauma material during Scene 1. Clinically, I knew that no matter what trauma-based thoughts, feelings, sensations, or images surfaced at this point, I would not put them into action. Instead, I would implement intervention modules for restoration, observation, and containment.

Trauma material did leak into this first scene. Tricia began to regress and ego state shift between victim and perpetrator roles as she put words to stories she had been told about herself as a child. When she began to enact the scene with the Colonel's baby, she showed aggression and hostility, compulsive action and dissociation.

Tricia accepted and worked well with both a containing double and a body double when prescribed to intervene on the flashbacks and body memories that had been triggered. Played by group members in therapeutic role assignments, these prescriptive roles benefited everyone. Tricia found roles of restoration and marked her observing ego roles, building a stable self-organization during Scene 1.

TSM Clinical Action Intervention Modules/Scene 1

The TSM intervention modules are described in the order in which they were implemented in Tricia's drama of conscious reexperiencing and developmental repair. The containing double is introduced. Restorative roles are discovered and enacted. The body double is added.

Creating the Containing Double

I introduced the clinical role of the containing double as the first TSM intervention module in Tricia's drama because our contract was for conscious reexperiencing of trauma-based scenes. I knew that she would need the support of this intervention module later in the drama so she would not get overwhelmed with dissociated feelings and unprocessed material from her trauma bubbles. I asked her to pick someone to be her containing double, using that terminology without much description because she already knew the intervention module well. When working with a protagonist who is unfamiliar with the TSM roles, I would have taken more time to explain the role according to the following definition.

Operational Definition. The number, frequency, and length of each containing double sequence varies in practice. Each intervention module, however, has been standardized for training and research (Hudgins & Drucker, 1998). There are three simple steps in completing the containing double intervention module:

    1) Speaking in first person, the CD makes a reflection of the process, content, affect, intensity, defense structures, et cetera, that the protagonist is experiencing in the moment.
    2) Still speaking in first person, the CD makes a statement that narratively labels the ability (of client, group, and/or team) to contain

and manage the reflected process, content, feeling, defense, etc., into conscious awareness. This containing statement does not negate or deny the reflection already made. Most importantly, it does not expand emotion, but contains trauma triggers with words and labels.

3)   Then, the CD anchors the reflection and containment into the here and now through time references, sensory data, and/or interpersonal connections. The CD communicates that, in the present moment, management of trauma symptoms is possible with the help of the group and the team.

The containing double is often played by a team member until the technique itself becomes integral to the norms of the group. Then the role can be prescribed as a therapeutic role assignment for a group member or chosen by the protagonist.

In this case, Tricia chose Susan, another group member, to be her CD and I clinically accepted that choice. I knew Susan had internalized her own containing double in the months she had been in a TSM group. Clinically, it would be good practice for her to help Tricia hold this prescriptive role when the trauma-based roles were enacted.

Although I prescribed the CD early, this prescriptive role intervention is not active during this first scene in Tricia's drama, in terms of production. Instead, the CD bonds through nonverbal empathy, which is built on during Scene 2 when there is increased experiencing of trauma-based roles. Later in the victim scene, the CD, along with the body double, became critical interventions during controlled regression.

Building the Restorative Roles

After establishing the containing double, I ask Tricia to choose more help for her drama today. I suggest people in her life. I mention spirituality. In this way, I am teaching that restorative roles are needed in all areas of life: personal, interpersonal, and transpersonal.

One of the first restorative roles that she spontaneously produces in her drama is that of "god—with a small g." This is a transpersonal strength and is quite relevant to anyone with a trauma history. Tricia starts out by saying she doesn't know what she believes in about God and then, when her body memories starts, she calls out, "oh God." As team leader I catch this spontaneous production of a restorative role. I ask her to pick someone to be the god of her understanding. She picks Peter, a TAE who she likes and feels safe with from a previous workshop. He takes on the role and speaks in the third person, talking to Tricia directly. Then I have Tricia role reverse with god. The role reversal continues until she experiences a sense of permission to do the work she came to do.

The restorative roles are completed when she picks a group member to be her courageous lion (personal strength), and says the group can be her interpersonal support. As team leader, I check off in my clinical director's mind that her restorative roles are now available, indicating that Tricia can face her trauma material without depleting herself further.

Finding the Sleeping-Awakening Child

After Tricia has her transpersonal strength with her in Scene 1, she spontaneously finds her sleeping-awakening child role in the doll she brought with her to the workshop. Without thinking, she picks up her doll and offers her to god. When this happens, I role reverse her so that she speaks from the role of god to say what role the doll represents. Clinically, I asked Tricia to label the doll's role from her transpersonal strength to increase the likelihood she would describe a positive self-representation, rather than that of victim. Tricia (as god) says that the doll represents a "precious child of god," and the sleeping-awakening child is introduced into the drama.

If I had asked her to pick a label for this doll from her own role, she was more likely to see her wounded child, which is contraindicated this early in the drama. This is what I mean by directing the drama clinically. I made decisions for role reversal in the service of my clinical goals for Tricia, not psychodramatic ones for production.

Establishing the Body Double

For the last intervention module of Scene 1, I ask Tricia to pick someone to be her body double. Since our clinical contract is to explore body memories, I assess that a body double will be needed. I know there are group members who can take on this role, so I ask her to pick anyone to be this role. I am hoping to save my auxiliaries for the victim and perpetrator roles that we know are to come. As with the CD, I prescribe the role early on—in Scene 1—so Tricia can bond with the person who she picks to play this role.

Since Andrea knew the BD well from her own recovery from anorexia, she didn't need any more explanation of this intervention module. This intervention module can also be expanded, however, according to the following definition.

Operational Definition.   The body double speaks in the first person and stands near the protagonist or group member. The BD takes on the nonverbal behavior and paralanguage qualities of the protagonist or group member. It can be introduced as follows:

> The body double is a part of yourself that accepts your body—that feels good about being in the physical world. A part of you that can accurately feel, express, and label your feelings, without getting emotionally triggered or overwhelmed.

As an experiential TSM intervention module, the body double includes the following steps:

1.   Speaking in first person, the body double moves into close physical proximity to the protagonist, feeling and sensing through his or her body into the body of the protagonist. The body double gives enough time for the experience to build into a more conscious expression of words.

2.   The body double puts words on positive body sensations to establish a connection to a physical vitality—a physical state of spontaneous learning. The body double does not go beyond this step unless the protagonist has established a connection to a nonverbal sense of positive body awareness. Until this state of vitality is sensed, the BD makes only containing statements. Once the protagonist is stable in body and mind, then the BD can take the next step in this intervention module.

3.   Still speaking in first person, the body doubles expands awareness of unconscious sensorimotor representations of trauma, and puts words to them. When no words are coming for unprocessed sensations and emotions, the body double puts a few words to a movement or a posture, for instance, "I wonder why I am clenching my fists?" The BD waits for a response and takes cues on which statements to follow up on in terms of nonverbal communication.

4.   Finally the body double gives permission and support for the protagonist to have full emotional expression, while maintaining the ability to express what is happening in one's body. The BD supports the protagonist through controlled regression and emotional catharsis and puts words to the trauma scenes so that they can be integrated into the body.

Similar to the containing double, the body double is often played by a trained team member until there is enough wisdom in group members' own body awareness to take on the role.

In Tricia's drama she chose Andrea for the BD and I supported this as a therapeutic role assignment. Andrea had done well with internalizing her own body double to contain her body memories, and could now eat regularly, if not a lot at each meal. Her body was beginning to be her friend again. I knew it would be a challenge for Andrea to hold this role in the face of Tricia's work on body memories, but thought she was up to it. I also knew if Andrea got stuck or overwhelmed in the role, I could have the AL support and coach her if needed.

Neither the CD nor the BD were very active during this first scene, but they were clinically indicated given the contract for conscious reexperiencing. The restorative roles were spontaneously produced. The transformative role of the sleeping-awakening child was concretized in the doll. God is played by a TAE. The observing ego was marked and available for role reversal, if needed, to maintain cognitive awareness through the cards used in the Friday night TSM structure of the workshop.

TEAM ROLES

During the prescriptive role scene, the TAEs begin to bond with group members. They sit next to people. They take on body double or containing double roles as directed by the assistant leader. The assistant leader accesses the individual needs in the group and prepares support for conscious reexperiencing of trauma-based roles for all. The TAES bring her information and she stores it as clinical knowledge for later use as needed. Having developed the prescriptive and transformative roles needed for conscious reexperiencing, the team is now ready to move into the first trauma-based scene in Tricia's drama. Scene 2 modifies primitive defenses in action and produces the change agent role.

SCENE 2: WORKING WITH DEFENSES IN ACTION

After the prescriptive role scene is completed, I clinically directed Tricia toward her trauma material to see what defenses and coping abilities would show up. Again, I am not following the protagonist into a trauma scene. I am clinically guiding her increased experiencing using the TSM principles of conscious reexperiencing: talk, observe, and witness. In this way the team can prevent uncontrolled regression and unconscious abreaction during Scene 2.

DIRECTOR'S SOLILOQUY

As Tricia and I start Scene 2, I ask her an open-ended question: "What do you see here?" This question invites her to project unconscious information into the circle of safe experiencing. I remind her that she has the help from her prescriptive roles to go into her body memories and trauma bubbles safely. She begins to allow herself to do that.

Tricia starts to relate stories she has been told about herself by her older sister. Body memories begin almost immediately. Her voice sounds like a little girl's. She starts to twist her clothes and turns away from her prescriptive doubles.

She briefly dissociates. She quickly regresses. She shows how she has identified with the aggressor and internalized this role. She hears herself use her father's words and voice. She unconsciously and compulsively acts out hatred and violence toward the Colonel's baby. She shifts ego states from child victim to father perpetrator.

I use the principles of conscious reexperiencing (described in chapters 7 and 8) to clinically direct Tricia's drama when she becomes triggered. When she starts to regress to a trauma scene, I direct her auxiliaries to increase production and use the principles to assess whether she can progress through the steps without further decompensation.

First, she must talk to us and tell us what she is going to enact with containment. Then she has to be able to observe and witness the scene without being triggered into uncontrolled regression. To help Tricia move into an observing role, I take on the prescriptive role of a keeper of defenses.

I role reverse her whenever she gets triggered into primitive defenses. I don't work to concretize and modify the defenses. I just role reverse her out of the roles that she was regressing into—the victim child and the internalized perpetrator roles—and put her in an adult observing role. I keep the defenses in place and note their rigidity to Tricia. I suggest that she could listen to her prescriptive roles and try something different.

Tricia found role reversal into her observing ego allowed her *to do something different.* From this clinical role, she was able to complete the principles of observing and witnessing the trauma-based scene. The OE role slowed her regression into a controlled, chosen pace. In addition, she could draw on the energy of her courageous lion, her god, and her prescriptive doubles from this therapeutic distance.

As TL, I directed the auxiliaries in these prescriptive roles to intervene with Tricia whenever she started to get defensive. The auxiliaries, trained team, and group members alike, took on the role of managing the prescribed roles of restoration, observation, and containment to help Tricia maintain conscious awareness at all times.

The auxiliaries managed the defenses. I clinically directed the auxiliaries. Tricia got to experience the ability to stay present to unprocessed trauma images and sensations that had haunted her for years. She could experience a state of spontaneous learning and put new words to old experience, as she kept moving her defenses aside to stay in the present moment.

Developmental repair happened when she was in her OE role, surrounded by her prescriptive roles. God said, "Stop, don't hurt that child," and adult Tricia could respond in a new manner. She had begun to internalize the transformative role of setting boundaries for herself in a new and healthy way.

The change agent role appeared and god protected and comforted Tricia as a 5 year old. In a spontaneous state of learning, she was able to let this new experience happen. Her defenses were set on the sidelines and she was connecting with herself in a new way. By the end of Scene 2, Tricia had found new words as well: she was a precious child of god who deserved to be cared for and loved.

TSM CLINICAL ACTION INTERVENTION MODULES/SCENE 2

Scene 2 introduces the transformative intervention module, the manager of healthy functioning. This module moves from the trauma-based role of the holder of defenses to the prescriptive role of the keeper of defenses, in the process of developing the transformative role of manager of healthy functioning.

Using the Body Double and Containing Double

These two roles are crucial throughout Scene 2. Together, working as a tag team, the body double and containing double follow each other with statements that produce containment of trauma material and defensive responses. Tricia does not get overwhelmed but is able to walk that fine line of accessing her dissociated feelings and unconscious compulsive actions, and being able to label them at the same time.

She doesn't have to resort to dissociation and other primitive defenses that block out her conscious awareness. Her courageous lion roars protectively in front of her when Tricia is in her OE role. She can safely watch herself as a 5-year-old child to see what connections the past has to her current symptoms of PTSD, body memories and flashbacks.

Her CD helps her to stay present and not become ashamed when she sees herself act compulsively. She can make sense of what she is seeing. Tricia says she was doing to the baby what was done to her. Her body double helps her connect visually with the group to stay in the here and now. The BD also helps her remain connected to her adult body state.

Building the Manager of Healthy Functioning

The manager of healthy functioning is the second transformative role that develops in Tricia's drama. By the end of Scene 2, Tricia has been able to let go of her primitive defense structure. She is able to stay present, connect with others, and create some new meaning from old trauma experiences. She has found her ability to manage her own internal processes and interpersonal connections differently. She is able to put words to previously unprocessed trauma bubbles.

As often happens, this role is never externalized in Tricia's drama. As mentioned, I take the prescriptive role of the keeper of the defenses for Tricia. The assistant leader performs that function for the group. Primitive defenses surface and the team intervenes. Gradually, Tricia learns how to manage her defenses with the help of her auxiliaries, and the keeper role becomes a manager of healthy functioning.

The defenses are still there, but she doesn't have to use them automatically. Instead she can listen to her CD and find words to say what is going on. She can feel her courage as the lion roars protectively in front of her. As with the other containing roles, the manger of healthy functioning intervention module can be further explained to clients and new team members using the following definition.

Operational Definition.   While this TSM advanced intervention module can seem complex in description, in experiential practice, these steps are easily implemented:

    1) The team leader identifies and labels primitive defenses that are surfacing in the face of trauma material. S/he asks the protagonist to mark them in action. Scarves, empty chairs, and people can all be used to concretize the defenses, depending on the level of active experiencing desired. As the team leader helps the protagonist externalize and label his or her defenses, the client begins to gain a sense of control over trauma patterns that are often experienced as automatic. This is the first step for the protagonist in working to modify defensive structures.

    2) The team leader asks the client to concretize the trauma-based role of the holder of defenses in order to externalize the rigidity of primitive defense structures. The TL teaches about the role of holder, commenting that primitive defenses are rigid and automatic. They are held in place, no matter whether they are needed or not. Then the protagonist picks someone to be the holder of defenses. So, now we have the defenses and the holder of defenses marked on the stage for observation.

    3) The third step in this intervention module is to resource the client with his or her prescriptive roles after marking the defenses and the holder of defenses role. As new spontaneity flows into the scene, the holder role begins to change and become less rigid. The TL directs the auxiliaries to talk directly to the protagonist to put action demands for new skills. The TL role reverses the protagonist into positive roles if the trauma-based roles of defenses and the holder become predominant in the interaction.

    4) Next the team leader introduces a new prescriptive role, that of the keeper of defenses. S/he role reverses the protagonist through the trauma-based roles of the holder and the defenses, and this new prescriptive role. Internal dialogues are externalized and enacted in

the here and now, so that new interventions can be made in old trauma patterns. This three-way spontaneous interaction gradually modifies the protagonist's use of primitive defenses. The holder role develops into the keeper of defenses role as the protagonist shows use of more positive ways to cope, i.e., to use a CD or a BD to stay present rather than dissociating. Now, the protagonist is able to hold trauma-based roles in awareness so observation and restoration can produce change.

5) As the creative interaction occurs between prescriptive, trauma-based and transformative roles, the protagonist finds new-found strengths and competencies. Clients experience that they do not need to rely on primitive defenses in the here and now, and new behaviors emerge. When the protagonist is able to stay in the present, connected to self and others, the transformative role of the manager of healthy functioning emerges and is demonstrated in action.

The above description shows how this intervention module can be concretized using auxiliaries, group or team members, to provide the interactions needed for the manager role to develop. This can also be achieved using empty chairs to hold the various roles in an individual session. However, in many cases, it is the team itself that holds the manager of healthy functioning role.

In Tricia's drama I held the manager function, directing the auxiliaries as clinically needed to maintain healthy functioning. The CD increased cognition when Tricia got emotionally triggered. The BD decreased dissociation so she could stay in her body, despite body memories. The courageous lion would give a roar every once in a while to quiet everyone. The OE put words to trauma-based actions from a safe therapeutic distance, maintaining her adult state.

By managing the auxiliaries I could adjust Tricia's level of experiencing so she could let go of her defenses safely. She no longer had to rigidly defend against thoughts and feelings from the past. We found the balance point in the present moment of the drama where she could observe, feel, and label what was happening without uncontrolled regression.

Finding the Change Agent Role

During this increased interaction among trauma-based and prescriptive roles related to defenses, the change agent role emerges. It is not a separate role in Tricia's drama, instead the transpersonal strength of god demonstrates the ability to stop the violence and produce change in action. In this case, Peter, a TAE, as "god" spontaneously stops the repetition of violence toward self. Instead, he offers comfort to the protagonist and in this way establishes the change agent. Only then, can the drama safely progress to active experiencing of trauma-based roles directly.

Developing the Sleeping-Awakening Child

In Scene 2, I role reversed Tricia into the role of the 5-year-old child, so she could experience developmental repair from this role. She is almost ready to consciously reexperience this child role as a trauma-based role, and I want her first experience of it to be positive. I want her to experience the energy of her sleeping-awakening child, joined with the conscious awareness of the wounded child, so that developmental repair can occur.

Prior to this role reversal by Tricia into her 5-year-old self, the sleeping-awakening child role has been held in her doll. This clinical intervention transfers the healing energy of repair from her doll to her own child role. Five-year-old Tricia talks to god. She lets go of her defenses. She takes god's hand, bringing her body and containing doubles with her. In role reversal to protagonist, Tricia cries and releases her shame. She discovers feelings of faith, trust, and hope. She connects with herself and others.

TEAM ROLES

As the drama spirals deeper into unconscious trauma bubbles, the team necessarily becomes more active to maintain support for conscious awareness. In addition to the description of my role as team leader, the other team roles can be highlighted in Scene 2.

Assistant Leader

Colette as AL held the keeper of defenses role for the group. She gathered people into clusters so that their changing feelings and ego states could be managed more readily. When a few people started dissociating in the face of the increasing hostility in Scene 2, she assigned Mark to be their CD to help them stay in their bodies. He helped them discriminate their triggers from what was happening in Tricia's story, so they could stay present and put words to what they were experiencing.

By the end of Scene 2, there were three clusters of group members in the observing space outside the circle of experiencing:

1)   a dissociated cluster with Mark/TAE acting as CD,
2)   an observing cluster that was taking notes, and
3)   a feeling group that was moving around the room with Vladimir as CD with them.

Trained Auxiliary Egos

The benefit of having trained auxiliary egos is evident in Tricia's drama. During Scene 1 they helped contain the group's energy. They found narrative labels for group members that began to be triggered. They provided support as needed.

I was able to ask Tricia to choose between Wendy and Ann, both team members, to play the victim role of the Colonel's baby. Ann played this crucial role so that a group member did not have to do so. This allowed Tricia the freedom to experience her compulsive energy without worrying about its impact on another group member. It also allowed the team to assess how people responded to the trauma-based roles surfacing spontaneously. Peter, another TAE, held the most important role for change in the drama so far. Because the god role had been spontaneously produced early in the drama, the team knew that it was a role that had the potential for healing.

As Tricia moved into witnessing the trauma scene, the team knew that the clinical goal was for the change agent role to emerge. A protector, a rescuer, a good mother or father, a compassionate god had to show up in the scene or we would not continue the contract further into conscious reexperiencing. With the final scene of developmental repair in the child role, Scene 2 is complete.

CONCLUSIONS

Tricia has successfully navigated the first three principles of conscious reexperiencing: talk, observe, and witness. Using her prescriptive roles, she has watched an unprocessed trauma memory and put new words to her experience. A change agent has emerged. The sleeping-awakening child is developing. She is now ready to move into conscious reexperiencing of the trauma-based roles, which is processed in chapter 10.

CHAPTER TEN

Enacting the Victim Role for Developmental Repair: Advanced Action Intervention Modules in Scenes 3–6

CHAPTER OVERVIEW

This chapter completes the clinical processing of Tricia's TSM drama of conscious reexperiencing with developmental repair. The final three principles of conscious reexperiencing—reenact, reexperience, and repair—safely guide controlled regression into the state dependent learning of trauma-based roles, in this case, the victim role.

As does the previous chapter, chapter 10 follows the intervention modules in Scenes 3–6 in the order in which they are presented in Tricia's drama (see chapter 8 for dialogue). Scenes 3 and 5 spiral into two separate unprocessed trauma scenes, while Scene 4 breaks the intensity with a return to observation and cognitive processing. The reader is able to see how the Therapeutic Spiral Model maintains the cognitive/emotional balance needed for conscious reexperiencing and expression of dissociated feelings.

This chapter also presents the TSM advanced action intervention module for safe enactment of all trauma-based roles, including victim, perpetrator, and abandoning authority. This step-by-step TSM structure teaches controlled regression and facilitates conscious abreaction when working with trauma bubbles. This structure moderates the pace as clinically needed for containment and observation.

SCENE 3: CONSCIOUS REEXPERIENCING OF THE VICTIM ROLE—THE COLONEL'S BABY

In Scene 3, Tricia is able to consciously explore a body memory that is triggered when she talks about herself as a child. She consciously reexperiences the role of the Colonel's baby for further exploration and finds it a screen memory. Following an affect bridge, she spirals to another memory, one of her father sexually abusing her. She finds accurate labels for her childhood experiences and puts accurate labels to unprocessed body memories.

DIRECTOR'S SOLILOQUY

As Tricia and I begin Scene 3, I am not sure what we will find. She is, after all, exploring unprocessed material from trauma bubbles. TSM clinical action structures create the container for this exploration, but the team does not know what will be discovered and expressed. As a clinician and team leader, what I do know is that Tricia is well resourced at this point in the drama. She is as safe as she can be, with prescriptive and transformative roles available to support her in the victim role. In TSM, the protagonist does not go back to the core trauma scene alone in a child role. Both the body and containing doubles will be beside her when she is ready to reverse roles into the victim role.

In this scene, Tricia follows the principle of reenactment and does a walk-through of her experience as the Colonel's baby. I assess that she is able to increase her experiencing of this role without setting off primitive defenses.

Next, we follow the principle of reexperiencing and move into the spontaneous production of the Colonel's baby role. Tricia lets herself regress to the state dependent learning that is stored in this victim role. She takes her prescriptive doubles with her, so she is not alone. I pace the regression to maintain a conscious level of active experiencing in the victim role. We can stop or start at any moment.

As she in is the role of the Colonel's baby, Tricia spontaneously and, most importantly, *consciously* follows an affect bridge between that scene and a body memory of being sexually abused by her father when she was 3 years old. She finds horror, terror, rage, and despair that have been held in trauma bubbles. She is able to express her dissociated feelings—with the help of her doubles and other auxiliaries. She finds new words to put her trauma memories to rest.

TSM ADVANCED INTERVENTION MODULES

Tricia walks the clinical line between increased experiencing of the victim role and maintaining her cognitive ability to put words to this new experience. The team and I hold the manager of healthy function as before. The auxiliaries help Tricia stay conscious and able to label what is happening in the here and now. There are no new intervention modules presented in this scene.

Using the Body and Containing Doubles for Controlled Regression

In Scene 3, these prescriptive roles are crucial to maintaining the safe pace of controlled regression and conscious expression of childhood feelings. With Tricia, they help contain and ground her in any role she takes, but especially when she moves into a trauma-based role. They are beside her when she is the role of the Colonel's baby.

As I witness her struggle to bring the past memory into present awareness, I see her ego state shifting before my eyes. She sounds like a scared little girl one minute, an angry, hostile adult the next. With her prescriptive doubles supporting her, Tricia is able to consciously reexperience the role of the Colonel's baby for exploration. She travels the affect bridge from this body memory to a fragment of another memory—of her own sexual abuse at age 3.

The containing double labels the coexisting states of self organization represented by the Colonel's baby, Tricia's 3-year-old self, the internalization of her father's voice, and the adult Tricia in this scene. The CD stabilizes the surplus reality of the multiple states of awareness by putting words to them. Tricia can have her feelings and tell us what they are at the same time.

The body double helps support controlled regression and conscious feelings in two ways. The BD provides a physical presence beside Tricia during ego state shifts that keeps her connected to a healthy state of nonverbal awareness. Through nonverbal empathy, the BD maintains the physical state of the adult ego.

The body double also put words to the dual sensations of the baby's body and the adult's body. This way, Tricia is able to embody multiple states of consciousness with simultaneous awareness. She finds words to describe her body memories. She makes the connections between the past and present.

Practicing the Change Agent Role

God, as the change agent, once again steps in during Scene 3 to help Tricia stay conscious and controlled in her regression. When she starts to become overwhelmed with her feelings and sensations, god calls out and brings her attention to his presence as a transpersonal resource for her to use to stabilize her ego state. The other restorative and transformative roles, established in Scene 1, continue to support Tricia in the present. Tricia ends Scene 3 having consciously reexperienced a body memory and put new words to it. She is safely reconnected to a sense of spirituality.

TEAM ROLES

As Tricia consciously reexperiences the victim role, both the assistant leader and the trained auxiliaries become more active to maintain containment and observation.

Assistant Leader

Colette/AL continues to work with the clusters of people she has set up during Scene 2. Mark (AE) holds the CD role for the dissociated group until most of them have moved from that cluster to the observing cluster. Group members can still find a therapeutic distance from the action outside the circle of experiencing without resorting, however, to the primitive defense of dissociation.

As I put Wendy in the victim role in this scene, Mark moves over to be the CD for the feelings group. Colette/AL coordinates these actions so that they do not disrupt the drama in the circle of experiencing. From time to time, she verbally lets me know what is happening so I can integrate the sub-scenes into the drama if I choose to do so for clinical reasons. At this point, I store the information for later use.

Trained Auxiliary Egos

One of the structures that makes this scene safe for controlled regression is the use of Ann (TAE) and Wendy (AE) in the trauma-based roles that hold both perpetrator and victim energy. Ann plays Tricia at 5 years old. This is the role that holds the perpetrator energy and needs to be modulated so it doesn't overwhelm Tricia. As team leader, I know I can count on Ann to walk that clinical edge with her dramatization of the role. She shows the compulsive energy, driven actions, and hostile voice tone that Tricia demonstrated in the last scene—while keeping it at an experiencing level that is manageable for the protagonist.

Tricia contracts to consciously regress to the Colonel's baby role. I put Wendy in as the doll, which is holding both sleeping-awakening child energy and the wounded child role at this point in the drama. This is the uncontained victim role in the scene, and I am glad to use an AE for this enactment.

Now the stage is set to work with the unclear self and object relations that are floating around between the doll, the Colonel's baby, Tricia's 5-year-old self, and her adult protagonist role. The next scene spirals up into observation and meaning making, so discrimination and stabilization can occur prior to exploring another trauma bubble.

SCENE 4: NARRATIVE LABELING AND WITNESSING OF THE CORE VICTIM ROLE

Scene 4 details a return to the earlier principles of conscious reexperiencing as we spiral directly to a second memory, a personal and core trauma scene. Tricia demonstrates that she can talk, observe, and witness the unprocessed information from the wounded child role that held the feelings of sexual abuse. A repair structure completes the action.

DIRECTOR'S SOLILOQUY

My clinical goal in Scene 4 is to have Tricia step into an observing role and tell us about what she remembers about her own core trauma scene. She has always carried visual memories of sexual abuse by both her father and godfather. This is not new information to Tricia.

What is new is being able to stay conscious and feel her feelings of horror, terror, rage, and despair in the face of these memories. In Scene 3 she felt the child state of the Colonel's baby. In this scene, she witnesses the body memory of her own victim role first from her adult state. Tricia observes what she has remembered before spiraling into conscious reexperiencing again.

As team leader, I want to externalize the trauma scene, so Tricia does not have to keep *unconsciously* reexperiencing it through body memories and flashbacks. Since she is shifting states among the adult protagonist role, the internalization of her father, and her child roles, I want to implement interventions of containment, observation, and restoration until she has stabilized her adult state.

This would have been an ideal place to implement the client role in the drama. As TL, I chose not to do so, because Tricia had already demonstrated the ability to hold more than one state in conscious awareness at the same time. Instead, I direct her to her OE role again. This role reversal increases active experiencing of her cognitive functions. We sit and watch the scene being reenacted in the circle of scarves. Once again, she is resourced by her courageous lion, god/the change agent, and her prescriptive doubles.

As we spiral into the past a second time, Tricia observes her father and her 3-year-old self in the same physical space as that of her 5-year-old self and the Colonel's baby. The object relations between victim and perpetrator roles remains the same in the original core trauma and in its representation toward the Colonel's baby. We follow that clinical connection in action.

To help stabilize self-organization, the team concretizes the internalized roles of victim and perpetrator. Wendy (AE) takes on the role of the "headless-wounded child." Mark (AE) is picked to play the sexually abusive father. Ann (TAE) moves into play the role of the doll in the drama. She now holds the role of the sleeping-awakening child in co-consciousness with the trauma-based victim role, played by Wendy.

I repeat what Tricia has said we will see—her father sexually abusing her when she is 3. I put the scene into action and she moves quickly from the principle of observation to witnessing. This time, she finds the change agent role inside herself. From her OE role, Tricia shouts, "No, I don't want it!" and stops the action in the drama, taking the role god played in Scenes 2 and 3. Tricia protects her faceless child and stops the cycle of violence from repeating. She claims her adult authority to make a difference in her own memories. God adds his voice to hers and together they tell her father to stop the abuse.

Then her feelings come through again, this time in her adult state. She grieves for her childhood pain and loss while she is held by her containing double, who fulfills the transformative role of good mother to self. Though the dialogue is not shown in chapter 8, this scene continues to develop for about 10 minutes, providing the container for her feelings and a strong sense of developmental repair. A group member spontaneously offers "Unconditional Love" and is brought into the circle by the AL.

TSM Advanced Action Intervention Modules

Scene 4 does not call for additional intervention modules. We use the OE and the other prescriptive and transformative roles to observe, witness, and change this core trauma memory, following the structure for experiencing the victim role in Scene 2.

Observing Ego Role for Observation and Witnessing

The first intervention in Scene 4 is to put Tricia into her observing ego role. From this role she follows the principles of conscious reexperiencing again. She tells us what we will see—her father sexually abusing her when she is three. She watches the impact on herself, the splitting of good and bad, at the time of the abuse. She finds new words to understand what happened to her at a very deep level. As she is in this role, I assess she can move deeper into reexperiencing of her own personal trauma scene.

Concretizing Splits in Self-Perception

As a clinician, I also want Tricia to observe the object relations that can be shown using experiential methods. I externalize her split self-representations by using Ann and Wendy in the separate child roles. Using two TAEs, one holds a positive image of self—the child of god with a face. Right next to it, I put the negative image of the self—the wounded, faceless child.

Ann was first put into the drama because she looked childlike and took the role of the child of god. She has played 5-year-old Tricia, trying to hurt the Colonel's baby. Now, she is assigned to play the baby who has a face. I am trying to enliven the sleeping-awakening child role with this role assignment. I want that healing energy to integrate the split self-organization.

Next, I assign Wendy the faceless baby role. She has held the unknown victim roles so far and this is another extension of that for her. I want this perception externalized to enable Tricia to see her terror and pain. Then she can decide what she needs to do to bring repair to the past scenes of trauma.

Tricia can now "see" how she has split her self-awareness in reaction to the original core trauma of sexual abuse. She has two self-representations: a child of god and a faceless child. This split has kept the feelings of childhood hidden from her, but it has also kept her away from her own spark of life. I sit with her and support her while she finds her spontaneity with the auxiliaries surrounding her.

This time, when she sees the abuse start, she immediately stops the scene. She sees her self as whole and acts on this perception. She intervenes immediately from the observing ego role and the change agent role develops further in her intrapsychic role atom.

Internalizing the Change Agent Role

In Scene 4, Tricia demonstrates that she has internalized the change agent role. In Scene 2 it was produced by a TAE in the role of god. It was again practiced by the TAE in Scene 3. Now, the change agent role is internally strengthened when Tricia immediately protects her younger self and stops the abuse. We know we can spiral deeper into conscious reexperiencing of her personal trauma role with safety and care.

TEAM ROLES

The main focus of the action trauma team in Scene 4 is to help the group to increase their roles of observation as well as the protagonist's capabilities for witnessing her trauma-based roles.

Assistant Leader

Colette/AL continues to work with the feelings that are in the group. Because this is a witnessing scene, she helps contain the feelings at a manageable level. She brings the observing and feeling clusters together and puts them into pairs. The observer supports the feelings so that they stay present but do not overwhelm the person having them.

Trained Auxiliary Egos

The core trauma scene was enacted by trained clinicians in the roles of victim and perpetrator. Tricia is able to watch the scene and the team does not need to worry about the auxiliaries being triggered in role. They know how to walk the clinical contract for increased experiencing, while maintaining the cognitive awareness needed to find new words for old stories.

Even if a team member does get triggered, the AL just moves in to help the team member contain his or her response. Ultimately, TAEs learn to use their own trauma responses in the service of the client. Later, in team meetings, TAEs express their feelings and get support to prevent secondary PTSD.

SCENE 5: CONSCIOUS REEXPERIENCING OF CORE VICTIM ROLE—TRICIA'S THREE-YEAR-OLD SELF

In Scene 5, Tricia consciously reexperiences a body memory of childhood sexual abuse for developmental repair. The TSM advanced action intervention module for the safe enactment of trauma-based roles is demonstrated, in this case, with the victim role. This experiential module provides simple clinical steps to control regression and promote conscious expression of feelings at the deepest levels of psychological healing.

DIRECTOR'S SOLILOQUY

Tricia is ready to make an informed decision about what she needs for her healing. Clinically, she has demonstrated she can witness her own core trauma scene and can interrupt the cycle of violence. Now, she can choose to consciously reexperience her 3-year-old child role to access state dependent learning.

I start this scene in a similar fashion to Scene 3. I invite her to project anything she sees internally into the circle of safe experiencing. We are, once again, concretizing her primary process in the here and now. I ask her what will bring repair to focus on healing, even as she explores a trauma-based scene.

Her doll continues to be a projection tool for her to externalize her surplus reality. She picks up the doll and sees an image of herself when she was called Rosalie, her family nickname as a child. She seems pleasantly surprised by this experience, and I predict to myself that it will emerge as her sleeping-awakening child.

To clarify, I ask her is it Rosalie with or without a face? Child of god or wounded child? I want to know what her self perception is at this point in the drama, having already worked to cognitively integrate the split self-representations in Scene 4 from a role of observation.

Tricia becomes overwhelmed with body memories. It as if the memories of Rosalie all of a sudden explode in her body awareness. She is triggered into uncontrolled regression and unconscious feelings begin bursting from trauma bubbles. It is at this point that the action trauma team is truly needed for clinical safety.

This team keeps Tricia on the edge between active and conscious experiencing of the unprocessed trauma memories, and creating new meanings to explain them in the here and now. Her CD helps her to find words to break the body memory's pull. Her body double claims her child body back, and keeps Tricia aware of her adult body at all times. Her courageous lion threatens to devour anyone who wants to hurt Tricia. She is safe as she gains a foothold and slows the regression to a manageable pace.

It is interesting to note that this team is in fact peopled by other group participants. Andrea is the body double, which she knows well from her recovery from anorexia. Susan plays the containing double, having internalized that role for herself in previous TSM work. They are the primary supports for controlled regression for Tricia, and they do an excellent job. Even without clinical training, group members can come together and form a healing team when using the Therapeutic Spiral Model (Baratka, 1994).

Tricia completes her contract to understand her body memories. In a co-conscious state (both adult and child) she states, "It is my body. It is my vagina. Maybe that is what my body memories were trying to tell me . . . this is my body. No one else can use it but me."

The final TSM intervention in Scene 5 takes place when I role reverse Tricia out of the experiential child role and back to her adult OE role. She observes the effect her body memory had on the organization of her intrapsychic role atom. Ann, who had been playing the sleeping-awakening child role, gets scared and has once again split off when the doll is thrown to the ground. She stands outside the circle of experiencing to demonstrate the split. The scene ends with the awakening child looking expectantly at Tricia for re-integration.

Wendy, as the wounded child, still sits in the middle of the experiencing space. She is covered by scarves. She is dissociated and abandoned. This externalization of the trauma scene concretizes the fragmentation and discarding of the wounded parts of self. We see the internal damage done by sexual abuse.

Tricia is able to see that the headless and wounded child is still in need of care. She feels the pull of light and love from the transformative role of the awakening child. Tricia affirms that she wants to find her face and we contract for a final scene, one of developmental repair.

TSM ADVANCED ACTION INTERVENTION MODULES

Scene 5 shows the spontaneous interaction among the auxiliaries taking different roles in Tricia's intrapsychic role atom. Together they provide the safety for controlled regression, so that Tricia quickly moves through the steps in the intervention module to enact the victim role. To complete the list of TSM interventions, this scene also includes a description of the client role, which was not used in this drama.

TSIRA in Action

Scene 5 demonstrates how the energy of spontaneity and creativity can develop a state of new learning. Working together—the roles of the CD and BD, the courageous lion, compassionate god, and unconditional love, create the perfect holding environment. Tricia consciously reexperiences her body memories in a safe, controlled, clinical structure for developmental repair.

She screamed, she yelled, her body released long dissociated sensations and feelings. Her mind stayed present with the help of her auxiliaries and the team. She was able to bring her past childhood trauma into the present moment of adult reality for change and healing. Witnessed and supported by the group, she was able to fully reexperience unprocessed trauma bubbles and find new endings in the here and now.

Structured Enactment of Victim and Perpetrator Roles

While Tricia was able to maintain controlled regression and conscious expression of dissociated feelings fairly easily, that is not always the case for a protagonist. For trauma survivors, triggers can come at unexpected times, in unpredictable ways. This TSM intervention module to enact trauma-based roles is a simple set of clinical directions to guide increased experiencing of victim, perpetrator, and abandoning authority roles. It follows the principles of conscious reexperiencing as noted.

Operational Definition.   These six clinical steps emerged out of practice with trauma survivors. Together with them, I find ways to control the pace of regression of trauma-based roles with experiential methods. The team leader or therapist directs the intervention module through these steps as clinically indicated to maintain the cognitive-emotional balance of TSM.

Step 1.   The protagonist verbally describes the trauma-based role to be enacted (talk). Team leader and protagonist stand a physical distance from the place where a TAE will take the trauma-based role (observe). This space can be further marked and contained by using an empty chair or a scarf or another object to represent the victim or perpetrator role. The protagonist speaks in third person to describe this role from a place of observation first.

For example, if I had needed to interrupt the regression with Tricia, I could have stopped the action and simply marked the role of her father with an empty chair. Taking the auxiliaries out decreases experiencing. Then, I could ask her to describe his role from the therapeutic distance of observation rather than through experiencing.

Step 2.   The team leader assigns a trained auxiliary ego (TAE) to take the trauma-based role without any additional spontaneity. The TAE begins to voice some of the things the protagonist described, but does not speak directly to the protagonist (observe).

Step 3.   The protagonist gives a "voice-over" for the trauma-based role from continued physical distance, but begins to speak in first person as victim, perpetrator, or abandoning authority directly. Gradually, the protagonist and team leader move physically closer to the TAE playing the trauma-based role. The protagonist gives words, affective tones, and nonverbal movements for this role from first person (reenact). S/he takes on the full spontaneity of the role, but remaining one step out of the physical space of the role (witness).

Step 4.   The protagonist role reverses and takes on the trauma-based role. The TAE playing this role steps aside and becomes the containing double for the protagonist in the trauma role. S/he helps the protagonist experience unprocessed information from this role in a safe and controlled pace (conscious reexperiencing).

In classical psychodrama, the protagonist would simply role reverse with the auxiliary that is playing the victim or perpetrator role. Thus, the protagonist would become "Mother" and the AE playing Mother would now stand in the role of protagonist. In TSM, I want to maintain stable object relations and not get the trauma-based roles any more mixed up in self-organization than they already are. This is the reason for the clinical action structure of the actual three-way role reversal using the CD as part of the action structure.

Step 5.   The auxiliary playing the CD or client role now steps into the protagonist space to be the reciprocal role to the protagonist, who is in the trauma-based role. In this structure, the protagonist is actively experiencing the trauma-based role with the support of a containing double, while connecting with a self-representation, not the image of the perpetrator. This action structure helps the client discriminate self/ other representations, rather than adding to the internal confusion.

Step 6.   This step involves classical role reversal between protagonist and all trauma-based roles. This step only happens after the protagonist has shown cognitive awareness and self-support. This advanced action intervention module guides controlled regression in TSM. It supports conscious abreaction. At any point in the sequence, a team leader can stop the action of the trauma-based role and stabilize the adult ego state before continuing the principles of conscious reexperiencing.

Client Role

This prescriptive role was not concretized in Tricia's drama because she was able to stay integrated as she progressed through the trauma-based roles in her drama. Her BD and CD were doing such a good job of containment, this additional role of observation was not needed.

The client role is prescribed when there is a need to increase observation beyond that of the observing ego role. It holds the executive ego position in the TSIRA. It sees all and knows all—and still keeps walking, one foot in front of the other, through the drama, no matter how hard it gets.

TEAM ROLES

It is during the conscious reexperiencing of core trauma scenes such as Scene 5 that the beauty of an action trauma team can truly be appreciated.

Assistant Leader

Colette/AL is quite busy during this core scene of conscious reexperiencing. All her trained team members are in the protagonist scene. The good thing about that is that she knows the trauma scene will be well managed. It does, however, leave her to manage the rest of the group without team support.

There is much rage in the group. As Tricia claims her child body back, the group is mobilized to express their own anger. Colette gets the people who are feeling angry together and creates a "stomping dance" they can do. They stomp around the room, yelling at Mark who holds the perpetrator role: "I am stronger than you now. I won't let you hurt me anymore."

Two people remain outside of the action, crouched in terror together as they watch Tricia reexperience her body memories of sexual abuse. Colette role reverses them into their observing ego cards and warms them up to cognitive processing. She asks: "What do you see? Is Tricia in her adult or child state? What is happening with her awakening child? Did you see her split off because it got too intense? You can watch from this safe place and not need to split off from yourself, OK?" She puts on her psychodramatic skates and moves around the group, integrating the energy of all into the whole of Tricia's drama with skill and precision.

Trained Auxiliary Egos

As previously noted, the trauma scene is enacted with trained auxiliaries in all roles. Mark is playing the perpetrating father. Wendy holds the wounded child. Ann acts out the splitting and need for integration of the awakening child. As TL, I know I can trust that each of the TAEs will walk the therapeutic line of increasing experiencing of trauma roles, while maintaining the cognitive ability to label what is happening.

If they do get triggered, as does Wendy in particular, they bring their responses to the drama to the team meeting, as described in the next chapter.

SCENE 6: DEVELOPMENTAL REPAIR

Tricia has consciously reexperienced two levels of trauma-based roles in her TSM drama. She regressed into the victim role of the Colonel's baby. She went further and spiraled into the role of her own 3-year-old self who was being sexually abused. Scene 6 details the developmental repair that spontaneously happened, creating a life-affirming ending to a rich TSM drama.

DIRECTOR'S SOLILOQUY

In this final scene, I am focused on developmental repair. Tricia clearly states that she wants to find a face, a head, a personification of self, to complete this controlled regression into the past. In the aftermath of her body memory, she has her awakening child beckoning to her. Her doll is thrown out of the circle. The wounded child is still covered with the scarves of dissociation.

Ann, in the role of the awakening child puts spontaneous action demands on Tricia to accept and integrate this healing role into her life. I pick up on this clinical offering and direct Ann to continue to interact with Tricia. They connect with each other and pick up the doll together. Integration is happening as we watch.

I direct Tricia toward her wounded child so that full developmental repair can happen. Together they go to rescue and protect the faceless and headless child role that Wendy holds. They slowly remove the veils of dissociation and bring the wounded child into conscious interaction with the awakening child and the adult self.

One final role reversal is needed. I put Tricia in the role of her sleeping-awakening self. She lies on the floor next to the wounded child. She finds a moment of spontaneity and feels a body shift in her self awareness—now she has a head! Tricia experiences the somatic integration of her good/bad self-representations with joy and connection to others.

The back and forth interaction between Tricia, Ann, and Wendy in the roles of protagonist, awakening child, and wounded child complete the scene of developmental repair. I anchor in Tricia's new physical sensations—eye contact, the feeling of having a head, having her hair touched.

Ann does an incredible job of nudging Tricia to do the work of self-acceptance at the physical level of nonverbal empathy and communication. She asks to be found, but lets Tricia make the decisions about how much of this new experience to internalize. When Tricia still seems a little bit shaky, I welcome the interpersonal anchoring offered by Andrea, who has played her body double. She brings a mirror to Tricia, so she can see the light shining from her transformed face. You can feel the healing in this room. Tricia, the group, the team—we are all held in the light. This scene ends as various group and team members come up to affirm the changes in Tricia, so they can be anchored in the future.

TSM ADVANCED INTERVENTION MODULES

As can be expected, there are no new intervention modules implemented during the final scene of developmental repair. Here, the auxiliaries work together to fully cocreate a true experience of healing for one and all.

Healing the Split Object Relations

To promote integration and repair of the split in self-representation shown in the last scene, I anchor the images and roles that seem to be floating around the room. To do this, I physically put Ann, who holds the awakening child projections, and Wendy, who holds the dissociated, wounded feelings, in similar proximity in the circle of safe experiencing. They lie on the floor next to each other, heads touching. One is smiling, beaming light and love, waiting to be accepted. The other is still disoriented, tender, a bit scared, and not sure what will happen.

This clinical enactment allows Tricia, from the integrated role of protagonist, to see both self-representations at the same time. She sees how she split to protect herself. She sees her wounded self, but she sees her vital self at the same time.

When I role reverse her into the sleeping-awakening self, she feels the experiential shift of integration happen. Tricia is able to experience the pieces of her split self blending together. Now, she can integrate information and feelings from the past into the present. She feels and labels the changes taking place.

At the interpersonal level, the group supports her new perceptions and reflects her beauty back to her. Tricia finds new meanings and they are anchored in the present scene with sharing from both group participants and team members.

TEAM ROLES

The team works together during this final scene to wind the drama to an orchestrated close.

Assistant Leader

During the repair scene, it is the AL's job to "de-role" the auxiliaries. Mark is no longer needed in his perpetrator role, so Colette draws him aside and asks him about himself: "How are you Mark? What did you experience? How was your role like your life? How is it different?" Colette helps her AE put words to his experience and fully de-role him from the perpetrator energy.

The AL also directs group members to connect with each other. Some people have expressed their anger and are spent. Others are watching the repair scene with respect and awe. Colette checks with each of them and makes sure they are connected to self and others as the drama ends.

Trained Auxiliary Egos

Wendy and Ann both hold the externalization of the split victim role in Tricia's role atom. I trust that they are working toward the same clinical goals as I am—repairing the split. Ann takes an active role in focusing Tricia's attention on the sensations and perceptions of healing. Wendy holds the dissociated role until the energy shifts.

CONCLUSIONS

This chapter completed the presentation of the 14 TSM clinical action intervention modules:

PRESCRIPTIVE ROLE INTERVENTION MODULES

1) Concretizing the observing ego
2) Establishing the client role
3) Building the restorative roles
4) Developing the body double
5) Using the containing double
6) Introducing the keeper of defenses

TRAUMA-BASED INTERVENTION MODULES

7) Meeting the holder of the defenses
8) Concretizing defenses in action
9) Safe enactment of victim, perpetrator, and abandoning authority roles

TRANSFORMATIONAL INTERVENTION MODULES

10) Finding the sleeping-awakening child
11) Creating the change agent
12) Living the manager of healthy functioning
13) Connecting with good enough others
14) Labeling a good enough spirituality

This book has now presented these interventions as well as the six unique clinical action structures of the Therapeutic Spiral Model:

1) The Therapeutic Spiral Image
2) The Action Trauma Team
3) The Trauma Survivor's Intrapsychic Role Atom
4) The Types of Reexperiencing Dramas
5) The Principles of Conscious Reexperiencing With Developmental Repair
6) Advanced Action Intervention Modules

Much thanks goes to Tricia for sharing her drama to demonstrate the healing power of this experiential model to treat PTSD.

PART FOUR

The Future With Trauma Survivors

The final section of this book (chapters 11 and 12) brings the Therapeutic Spiral Model home for practitioners. Chapter 11 discusses self-care and the prevention of secondary PTSD as part of the overview of using experiential methods with trauma survivors. Training and research are discussed.

Of timely importance, the final chapter discusses direct applications of the TSM to the recent disasters in the United States. As the model has developed, it has been successful in treating a wide rage of stressors that cause PTSD, from childhood abuse to acts of terror and war trauma. In the end, PTSD is the same everywhere. The TSM can be used for effective and rapid treatment both at the clinical level of intervention as well as within communities.

CHAPTER ELEVEN

Preventing Secondary Posttraumatic Stress Disorder in the Practitioner

CHAPTER OVERVIEW

As the reader has experienced in Tricia's drama, there is great joy in walking side by side with people seeking to heal from past trauma using the Therapeutic Spiral Model. Spiraling to the depths of despair and pain is rewarded with empowerment and connection. These are the moments that matter.

Unfortunately, all work with trauma survivors can be as exhausting and draining as it can be exhilarating and joyful. Experiential therapy carries additional risks to providers. It is more intense, and potentially more disturbing, to see, feel, and hear people's traumas concretized in the here and now, than to "talk about" a trauma with a client. This has the potential to create secondary posttraumatic stress.

Given the intensity of traumatic experiences, therapists, counselors, advocates, relief workers, friends, and family members, can all find themselves affected by the horror of what humans can do to each other (Remer, 2000). This chapter presents the TSM structures that were developed to prevent secondary PTSD with members of action trauma teams who work with trauma survivors.

Team meetings and "doodah management" are core components to the success of staying clear in the midst of the chaos and primary process material in trauma bubbles. Transference and countertransference reactions are identified as part of the structure for containment and clearing in TSM. Personal sharing promotes transparency, unconditional regard, and empathic bonding. This chapter also presents the TSM structure for concretizing projective identification to prevent unconscious acting out by the group or team members during a TSM trauma drama.

TEAM MEMBERS IN ACTION

I would like to further introduce the TSM practitioners who made up the action trauma team for Tricia's drama. They are typical of the people who practice the Therapeutic Spiral Model to treat trauma using experiential methods of change. In addition to myself as team leader, the following people were present.

Assistant Leader

Colette Harrison, B.A., held the assistant leader role in Tricia's drama. She is a full-time international TSM trainer and team leader, and is Project Coordinator for our work in South Africa. She is trained as an addictions counselor and trauma specialist and has worked in a variety of settings over 20 years of clinical practice. She is a trained psychodramatist through the Moreno Institute and the accreditation program at Therapeutic Spiral International.

Throughout the year, Colette adds her voice to an international choir—One Human Family Workshops, Inc., a nonprofit organization. She travels the world to sing to promote racial unity and develop models of reconciliation. She does have a history of personal trauma from sexual abuse, alcoholism, and addiction to pain medication, which she shares readily in person. She is a valuable member of any action team!

Trained Auxiliary Egos

Ann is a TSM trained auxiliary ego, as well as an accredited assistant leader. In Tricia's drama and those of others, she often holds the TAE role because she likes the freedom of being the team member who "gets to enact the roles, rather than assess the roles."

She is a licensed clinical social worker who works part-time in private practice in a Midwestern university town. She is married and the mother of two daughters, aged 9 and 12 at the time of Tricia's drama. She brings commitment, love, and service to her role as an action team member. She participates on 4–6 TSM action trauma teams per year as part of her flexible schedule in private practice.

Peter is the other TAE in Tricia's drama. He represents participation on TSM action trauma teams by men and women in the business field.

He studied psychodrama as it applies to organizations in Australia for 3 years out of personal interest and has received TSM clinical training. He is an accredited TAE and now participates on two to four TSM teams a year.

While Peter does not have a trauma history (other than a divorce), he is involved on TSM action trauma teams because it gives him an opportunity to "give back to others." Working in large, international companies as an accountant, he finds that his work as a trained auxiliary ego on quarterly TSM teams gives him a chance to know himself and the world in a better way.

AUXILIARY EGOS IN TRAINING

Most TSM teams have at least one team member in training. Supervised practice is a core component of learning the Therapeutic Spiral Model and is achieved through team practicums while in training. These AEs are representative of practitioners training in TSM at this level of accreditation. (See Appendix C for accreditation standards.)

Wendy is a clinical social worker who directs a women's shelter in a large mid-Atlantic city in the United States. She works full time and is a single mother. She has a personal history of long-term sexual abuse as a child and domestic violence as an adult. Wendy had been in ongoing TSM training for 1 year at the time of Tricia's drama.

Mark is a psychiatric resident at a New York City hospital. He was born in Israel and is completing his training in the United States. His parents were survivors of the holocaust, where he lost two generations of family members. He had participated in two quarterly training sessions in the Therapeutic Spiral Model given by the psychiatry department at a teaching hospital in New York City before Tricia's drama.

These are the people and the roles of the action trauma team that helped Tricia enact her drama of conscious reexperiencing and developmental repair. This chapter now presents the TSM structures to keep team members well resourced when doing this intense work with trauma survivors.

TEAM STRUCTURES TO PREVENT SECONDARY PTSD

The structure of having an action trauma team is, in itself, a counterbalance to the stress of practice with trauma survivors. The simple fact that the practitioner is not alone makes the work much easier. It is a help if one's own trauma history is reactivated or a team member experiences strong countertransference reactions. In the Therapeutic Spiral Model, team members can have their own personal processes, in the privacy of team meetings that provide a safe container for processing, debriefing, consultation, and supervision. "Doodah management," which is described later in this chapter, helps keep interpersonal conflicts to a minimum. The final TSM structure to prevent secondary PTSD for team members is to learn how to identify and enact projective identifications (PIs). These team structures are designed to maximize healthy functioning at both individual and team levels.

TEAM MEETINGS

For each and every TSM workshop, group, or personal psychodrama, there is both a pre- and post-session team meeting to support the providers in this trauma work. When weekend or residential workshops are part of the plan, team meetings are scheduled at the beginning and end of each day, as well as a brief meeting held over lunch. Team meetings also provide a place for team members to resource themselves with prescriptive roles and even, if necessary, scenes of developmental repair. These meetings allow the team to clear any interpersonal difficulties that arise and to plan the next session in the here and now.

Pre-Session Team Meetings

Pre-session team meetings give team members a chance to warm up together. They share personal strengths and vulnerabilities, make connections with each other, and mark any areas of containment that are needed. This simple pre-session structure takes between 1 and 2 hours. At the end of the meeting, the team is well contained, well connected, and ready to be of service to the clients.

Before Tricia's session, Wendy shared that she felt able to take on any role, and would like to try a victim role. This was her third TAE practicum experience on a Therapeutic Spiral team. She had learned to identify and contain several triggers that could set off her own trauma history during a drama. Now, she wanted to test out her skills at a trauma-based role, one of the requirements for accreditation as a trained auxiliary ego in TSM.

This pre-session sharing gave me permission (as team leader) to ask her to play the core victim role in Tricia's drama. She did get dissociated under the veil of scarves and it was good to know in advance that she wanted to work with this when it showed up. Otherwise, I may have taken her out of the role when she became triggered into primitive defenses.

During the action, Colette, as AL, kept checking in with Wendy while she was in the victim roles. At one point, she took the veils off, fanned her face, and gave her a drink of water. Wendy found she could walk the line between her own triggers and the enactment of an intense victim role—with support from the AL.

Because Mark was a new team member to me, I chose to share my own personal history of childhood sexual abuse before the workshop started. I shared with him that I had been adopted at birth into an extended family that was powerful and wealthy—and abusive and alcoholic. I told him the development of the Therapeutic Spiral Model came out of my own recovery from PTSD, along with my training as a clinical psychologist and certified psychodrama trainer (the three strands of the model).

Next, the team reviewed the clients and their referral and intake information. The group had a variety of traumatic experiences. Several themes were apparent: the generational transmission of trauma, feelings of rage and despair, and the desire to live free of the past.

As team leader, I noted out loud a possible parallel process that Mark might get stuck in. Mark had reported that his wife had been seeing him in a "perpetrator role" lately. She saw him as self centered, driven to succeed, and uncaring. She said he didn't have time for his family and that the kids were suffering. We knew it was likely that he would be picked to play a perpetrator role. When this happened, Colette helped him stay contained, knowing his own situation was so fresh in his mind. She supported him with brief "hit and run" containing double statements as needed.

Post-Session Team Meetings

Post-session team meetings share a similar format to pre-session meetings with personal check-in and sharing of the impact of the drama. In addition, there are added emphases on

- de-roling from victim, perpetrator, and abandoning authority roles,
- use of the prescriptive roles to clear personal difficulties *prior* to any interpersonal encounters among team members, and/or
- referral for further supervision or therapy as needed.

The debriefing process takes about 1 1/2 to 2 hours, depending on the number of team members. If team members are not completely comfortable at this point, issues are marked for therapy or supervision.

De-Roling. In the post-session meeting following Tricia's drama, Wendy needed help in de-roling from the victim roles she had played. She had felt triggered into her own wounded child and her primitive defenses against these feelings. She said she felt dissociated and alone.

First, I directed each team member to give her positive feedback for the work she did in the victim role, so that her mind would become engaged in the here and now. Next, I set up a nurturing hold where Ann could support Wendy while she had her feelings. Wendy let herself cry as long as she needed. She accepted the comfort of the team as good mother.

Cognitively, it made sense that this action was a needed completion, following Tricia's drama. There had been no mother available to Tricia, even in the conscious reexperiencing scene where her doubles and other supportive auxiliaries provided the psychological holding needed. Thus, the transformative role of good mother emerged in the team meeting as a final scene in the weekend.

Mark also needed help de-roling from playing the perpetrator role. As with Wendy, the team first gave him positive feedback on his skill level in the perpetrator role to provide a cognitive frame for further intervention. Then, as team leader, I directed him to put two chairs back to back. One chair represented Mark as he is today. The other represented the abusive father he played in Tricia's drama. He was asked to make statements about how he was different from the role he had played. Each time he clarified a difference, the chairs moved farther apart.

At the end of this action sequence, he sat in his chair and was asked to say anything he wanted to the empty chair that represented the father. He said,

> I am very different from you. I have struggled with my temper and with my own self-centered needs. I make different choices than you did. I love and protect my kids. Maybe I'm not home as much as I would like, but I would never hurt them like you hurt Tricia . . . ah . . . Rosalie.

Personal Sharing. In many ways, providing a clinical structure for personal sharing among team members is the essence of care in the Therapeutic Spiral Model. It provides a safe place for team members to share what is really going on, so there is no need to hide or compartmentalize personal and professional experiences. The rule of no shame, no blame applies to the team as well as to the clients.

As team leader, I set a tone that lets team members know they can share their vulnerabilities, as evidenced by my pre-session sharing with Mark. At the end of Tricia's drama, I shared with the group that while I had been sexually abused by more than one family member also, the abuse by my father had been the most difficult to reconcile. I both idealized him and hated him as I grew up. As an adult, I grieved over "being special," when I came to understand that meant I was also abused. I told the group, "today, I feel like a normal person and it's wonderful!"

"DOODAH" MANAGEMENT

The term "doodah management" was coined by an intern working with TSM trainer Mario Cossa, to learn the model as it applies to adolescents. For all people, this term "refers to the need for members of action trauma teams to learn to recognize, share, and work with awareness about the interaction of personal and trauma based material among team members" (Cossa, 1999, p. 1). Given that many action trauma team members have their own personal history of trauma, doodah management puts some humor into what can be, at times, tense moments on the team. Transference, countertransference, and projective identification can all stir up doodahs, making people reactive to each other.

Transference

The TSM works from a developmental perspective concerning transference. Transference is seen as a normal psychological process that helps people sort out his/her self-image from those of others. They are bound to occur in TSM dramas, so team members are clinically trained to work with transferences as they arise.

In Tricia's drama, I made some directing decisions based on transference. Because Wendy had a history of sexual trauma, I thought Tricia could easily transfer the role of her wounded child onto her. Wendy did, in fact, hold that role and the energy of the transference well. Tricia was able to witness her depleted, dissociated, wounded self and connect her with the sleeping-awakening child for transformation and healing.

Tricia picked Ann to play the role of her doll, and its representation as a precious child of god. She said she looked childlike, in a positive, innocent way. Throughout the drama I used this positive transference to Ann as a thread pulling through the various role reversals of the victim state. In the final scenes, self-representations of both good and bad integrated and merged into a vision of beauty and wholeness.

Countertransference

This is a doodah that is expected on TSM action trauma teams. Team members cannot witness the horror of trauma scenes and be unaffected. Part of debriefing is to share personal responses and to identify which issues were triggered during a TSM drama. This is called countertransference.

When narrative labeling is not enough to contain the countertransference, the TL may lead the team member in some clearing work. Had Mark not been able to complete his de-roling from the perpetrator role by the action structure detailed a few paragraphs ago, we could have worked at a deeper level. I could have asked him who it was that sat in the perpetrator chair for him. Who had passed the family legacy of struggle, despair, and ultimately death on to him? Then Mark could have dialogued with his own personal trauma-based roles for developmental repair.

PROJECTIVE IDENTIFICATION INTERVENTION MODULE

A final step in preventing secondary PTSD is to learn how to work with projective identification as a team intervention. Projective identification, as mentioned in chapter 5, is a normal developmental stage where people learn to moderate their affect through interactions with others (Schore, 1997). This intervention module involves use of a TAE to enact the projective identification or to be the CD to a client who is spontaneously acting it out.

Operational Definition

1) The team member begins by putting words to the experience of picking up a PI to bring it into conscious awareness.

2) The director and AL agree that the PI should be introduced into the trauma scene the protagonist is enacting. The TL directs the protagonist's attention to the role the team member is holding, for instance, shame, and asks whether this role belongs in the drama. If the protagonist answers yes, the TL chooses how to bring the role into the session. For example, the feeling of sadness can be brought into someone's drama in the role of a grieving mother or a caring spouse. Then the protagonist would have a chance to see if this feeling is, in fact, his or hers in the present moment.

3) Interaction must be increased to integrate PIs into the action. If the protagonist does not identify with the spontaneous PI, then a dialogue between the protagonist and auxiliary can finish the interaction, or a role reversal may extend it. When the protagonist role reverses with the PI, s/he gets an experiential awareness of the role and whether the feeling belongs in the drama. It is at this point that a PI can offer valuable experiential information to the protagonist. Is it his shame? Is it her rage? Through spontaneous interaction and role reversals, the protagonist becomes aware of new feelings and can choose how and when to express them.

To end this chapter on preventing PTSD, I want to share with the readers the song that the TSM trainer, Mario Cossa, wrote to add some humor to the process of doodah management.

THE DOODAH SONG

Lyrics by Mario Cossa (2000); sung to the tune of *Camptown Races*

If in your organization things are going wrong—doo dahs, doo dahs. You try to work things out but they don't last for long—doodahs could be at play.

Chorus: They can make you fight. They can ruin your day. Mountains made from molehills are a real good sign doodahs are at play.

You make a simple comment. Someone snaps a sharp retort—doodah, doodah. Faces getting long and tempers getting short—doodahs could be at play.

(Repeat chorus)

I'll project on you and you project on me—doodahs, doodahs. Sometimes it's hard to tell what is reality. Doodahs could be at play.

(Repeat chorus)

CONCLUSIONS

This chapter shows the importance of resourcing the providers who work with trauma survivors. Trauma work is demanding work. It has been known to push any and all unresolved issues that practitioners have. In the Therapeutic Spiral Model, team meetings, doodah management, and working with projective identifications provide the container for team members to stay healthy and whole doing this intense work.

CHAPTER TWELVE

The Future of Action Methods With Trauma Survivors

CHAPTER OVERVIEW

In the last 6 months, people have understood the link between traumatic stress and their own functioning in ways that this book could never have conveyed. Some of you, even those without a previous trauma history, may have identified symptoms similar to those of PTSD in your own life, following the attacks on the World Trade Center, the Pentagon, and the presence of anthrax found in postal mail. Hopefully, most of you have found experiential methods to begin using with your clients who are diagnosed with PTSD and other stress-induced disorders.

It is my conclusion that experiential methods are a treatment of choice for trauma survivors, when anchored in clinical theory and practice, as in the Therapeutic Spiral Model. The contents of this book summarize the accumulated body of knowledge on the impact of trauma demonstrated in the right-brained, nonverbal, and emotional symptoms of PTSD. This book ends as it started, by prescribing the Therapeutic Spiral Model to treat PTSD in action. When clinically guided, the modified psychodrama interventions detailed in this book greatly enhance change for trauma survivors. TSM increases treatment effectiveness and reduces the time needed to work through debilitating problems such as flashbacks, body memories, and nightmares. Tricia's drama showed the power of the model, along with the containment needed for safety.

This final chapter takes a look into the future of action methods to treat PTSD. Research, training, practical applications, and guiding visions all interweave to create an abundance of hope for people affected by trauma.

RESEARCH: THE PATH TO THE FUTURE

Every book in psychology and psychotherapy ends with the adage that more research is needed, and that is equally true in the case of the Therapeutic Spiral Model. In the past 10 years, experiential therapy has come of age. As Elliott, Greenberg, and Lietaer (2002) state in the new 5th edition of the *Handbook of Psychotherapy and Behavior Change,*

> In particular, experiential treatments have been found to be effective with depression, anxiety and trauma, as well as to have possible physical health benefits and applicability to clients with severe problems. (p. 12)

The Therapeutic Spiral Model is one such experiential treatment, one that is effective with trauma and PTSD. Clients have acclaimed the model for over 15 years. Self-reports and therapist reports show high levels of improvement in clients following a *Surviving Spirits or Trauma and Recovery workshop.* Research efforts are beginning.

As reported, a single case study (Hudgins, Drucker, & Metcalf, 2000) showed that the containing double significantly reduced dissociation and general trauma symptoms for a woman diagnosed with PTSD and having difficulties with body memories. Chapter 2 listed additional studies indicating that psychodrama and experiential therapy are effective with trauma survivors.

The next action step in TSM research is a planned international collaborative study, which is in its preliminary stages with TSM practitioners in Australia, Canada, England, South Africa, and the United States. Practitioners in training will conduct a 6-session containing double protocol with a minimum of two clients with PTSD over the course of the next year. The purpose of this investigation is to replicate the original study and to expand the testing of the containing double. Because TSM is an experiential method, it is hypothesized that the containing double will prove useful across cultures, at least in this case, in those that speak English.

CROSS-CULTURAL ADAPTATIONS

Action trauma teams versed in the Therapeutic Spiral Model have met the challenges of working in over 12 countries, some which did not speak English, in the last 7 years. This work has proven that a solid clinical framework that offers containment and narrative labeling to traumas is effective across populations and cultures. Using experiential methods actually bridges many of the gaps in communication between people of different languages and cultures. The body talks the same language when it comes to feelings. Cultures may frame the experience of emotion, but cannot disguise it as a basic commonality among humans. For many people in many cultures, seeing a trauma reenacted can change a worldview, whereas words might only lead to a quagmire. We will continue to conduct research to find support that is more than words as well.

TRAINING IN EXPERIENTIAL PSYCHOTHERAPY

As noted, it is a premise of TSM that practitioners need to be highly trained both in the principles of clinical practice and the expert use of experiential methods to work with trauma survivors. I hope this book has demonstrated how powerful the Therapeutic Spiral Model can be to treat trauma. Now, I want to emphasize the need for advanced training to do such work in a safe and effective way.

Appendix C describes the postgraduate training program that leads to accreditation in the Therapeutic Spiral Model. As all good clinical training programs do, it includes theory, practice, live supervision, and research. There is also a national certification process in psychodrama, sociometry, and group psychotherapy (ABE, 1982) in the United States. It has been adopted in Australia, New Zealand, England, Turkey, and other countries as a standard of training. The Association of Experiential Therapists also offers a national certification in action methods, that is local to the United States.

No matter what route is chosen, training to work with trauma survivors must be extensive, careful, and steady. This is a vulnerable population, wanting to trust, yet fearing to do so. Competent practice is a mandate of the call for action methods as a treatment of choice with trauma survivors, to prevent re-traumatization with these powerful methods.

Self-Care to Prevent Secondary PTSD

When working with the intensity of trauma day after day, it is important to practice an abundance of self-care activities to prevent secondary

PTSD, which can affect competent practice. It is hard enough to reach into the depths of your own being to witness the horror and terror others have experienced when one is feeling restored and renewed. It is almost impossible to do so when the practitioner is exhausted, overworked, and burned out.

Working in a collaborative team provides for self-care by its structure alone. TSM teams provide a structure that includes personal sharing, team meetings, and doodah management. All are designed to help prevent secondary PTSD. Team members support each other. They create a safe place to share vulnerabilities and draw on shared strengths. Most of all, colleagues share the experiences of walking through trauma. They are not alone with the terror, horror, despair, and rage of trauma. They are held in the container of the action trauma team.

When a team is not available, supervision can provide a personal support team for the practitioner working with trauma survivors. Supervision is required as part of most clinical training programs and is even more important when using experiential methods. Psychologically, supervision provides the container for the practitioner to identify and process his or her own trauma responses. It also improves clinical skill at directing trauma survivors safely. Of course, practitioners need to be willing to attend to their own psychological needs through personal therapy as needed.

Additional self-care programs that team members suggest include massage therapy, exercise, yoga, 12-step groups, church, and time with family. There are many ways to stay resourced and clear in work with trauma survivors. It just takes the commitment to do it as part of providing ongoing trauma services to people.

PRACTICAL APPLICATIONS: BUILDING ACTION TRAUMA TEAMS

In the years since the first *Surviving Spirits* workshop, Therapeutic Spiral International, the nonprofit organization I started, has sponsored action trauma teams in over a dozen countries. The Director of Training at TSI assigns team members to action trauma teams according to their expertise, geographical location, and availability. The clinical applications of the TSM have expanded with the interest of team members, as they learned the theory and methods of TSM and applied them to their own areas of interest. Because the Therapeutic Spiral Model is experiential, practitioners complete practicums to demonstrate competency with the model in the various team roles. This becomes a cocreative process of integrating areas of interest, present expert skills, and the new skills of TSM. In many cases, it has resulted in additional practical applications of the Therapeutic Spiral Model in action.

ADDICTION MEDICINE

In the past 2 years, the model has been adapted to work with alcoholism and addiction (drugs, sex, relationships), by an addictionologist in Canada. As he built an action trauma team for his private practice, this doctor found ways to use the power of 12-step groups within the clinical effectiveness of the Therapeutic Spiral Model.

Clients in these groups welcomed the chance to enact their "higher power" and make more conscious contact with the God of their understanding. Group members enacted the support of home groups and supported protagonists in their recovery. The power of the 12-step program was brought into the here and now to be used as interventions in TSM.

It is a perfect match, TSM and addictions, given the belief in both systems that spirituality is core to change. TSM gives practitioners of addiction medicine the tools to concretize the abstract qualities of a higher power, as well as provide behavioral rehearsal for relapse prevention. I am sure that this area of application will continue to expand.

EATING DISORDERS

Kathy Metcalf, LCSW, PAT, and Colleen Baratka, MA, TEP, of Baltimore and Philadelphia respectively, are TSM trainers and team leaders who focus on healing eating disorders. Together with a nutritionist, bodyworker, and massage therapist, they focus on concretizing the body double and teaching the physical state of spontaneous learning to people suffering from anorexia, bulimia, and compulsive overeating. Client reports provide great encouragement for this application.

WORKING WITH ADOLESCENTS

Mario Cossa, MA, RDT/MT, TEP, and Kamala Burden, MA, ADTR, RDT, of Keene, New Hampshire, have applied the TSM to children and adolescents. They found the need for differential interventions, based on age and psychological development, to be crucial with this population. Cossa created "Dragodrama" (2002) and integrated much of TSM theory into his own model of working with at-risk teenagers. His action trauma team is made up of clinicians who specialize in working with children and adolescents.

While the TSM started out as a method of experiential psychotherapy for trauma survivors, it has also been used in educational and community settings. Since 911, the TSM has been used to debrief large groups of first-response teams in NYC and to work in the postconflict environments of Northern Ireland and South Africa. In all cases, the TSM has been adapted to the different challenges met by large groups that know each other and will continue to work together in community long intervention by TSM practitioners.

The primary differences when using TSM in nonclinical settings relate to questions of history, self-disclosure, boundaries, and goals of intervention. In community settings it is enough to educate people about PTSD and bring them in contact with forgotten strengths or healing interpersonal wounds among members. In this way, the TSM still follows the clinical map of the TSIRA and uses the advanced action interventions, but finds a level of comfort for practitioners that does not overexpose them to their family, friends, and colleagues. These boundaries are most important for safety in a community setting.

Each practitioner who builds a local action trauma team applies it to the populations and problems they work with in their practices. In this way, TSM reaches the most people. After all, TSM is not a rigid model, but a clinical model that can be flexibly adapted to treat PTSD from any number of causes.

GUIDING VISIONS

Many people have called me a visionary, and the Therapeutic Spiral Model prophetic, especially since September 11th, 2001. In this book, however, I have tried to bring it all "down to earth." I have anchored the model in its theoretical foundations and the experiential principles of change. I have detailed 6 unique clinical action structures and 14 advanced intervention modules to guide experiential practice with trauma survivors. Tricia has shared her story so that readers can see the model in action.

THE LONGEST JOURNEY

I share with J. L. Moreno (1953) the vision that "A truly therapeutic procedure cannot have less an objective than the whole of (hu)-mankind" (p. 3). One of the greatest gifts of classical psychodrama is that in it, the spiritual aspects of life are presented as core to healing. Moreno (1920) believed each person was a "godhead," many decades before the "god within" became a fashionable secular belief in Western culture. All psychodrama techniques were originally developed to increase spontaneity and creativity, and in that way, reach the godhead (Moreno, 1973).

It is through this added dimension that experiential therapies can truly make a difference in the world. Recently, a few psychodramatists have been more directly addressing the psychospiritual side of healing (Miller, 2000; Winters, 2000). Transpersonal psychology is beginning to be recognized.

When working with trauma survivors, people who have actually experienced the worst of life, attention must be paid to their spiritual healing as well as to their physical, psychological, and emotional health. Only when the whole person is treated can the wounds of the past stop being passed on to new generations.

CONCLUSIONS

The introduction to the book presented a brief description of the elements of the TSM:

1)   *Client-friendly constructs of experiential self-organization for trauma survivors.* More than one survivor has said that the images of the therapeutic and trauma spirals have become a lifeline to them in times of body memories, flashbacks, and ego state shifts. They have readily embraced the construct of trauma bubbles. My hope is that these images have given practitioners an easy way to communicate with their clients, often at times when it is hard to find words.

2)   *Clear clinical action structures for safe experiential psychodramatic practice with trauma survivors.* This book presented 6 TSM clinical action structures that modify classical psychodrama techniques with trauma survivors. These structures utilize action methods and are guided from a clinician's eye. Tricia's drama demonstrated the use

of all the clinical action structures to consciously reexperience core trauma scenes for developmental repair. The reader witnessed controlled regression with the support of these clinical action structures.

3) *Advanced action intervention modules for containment, expression, repair, and integration of unprocessed trauma material.* In the clinical processing of Tricia's drama I described the modified psychodrama methods the reader saw in action. Fourteen action intervention modules were detailed, some with operational definitions for research and training. These advanced intervention modules concretize and enact the TSIRA's prescriptive, trauma-based, and transformative roles.

This book has brought together theory, research, and practice to illustrate the Therapeutic Spiral Model as a method of choice to treat trauma survivors.

POSTSCRIPT

My favorite epigram from J. L. Moreno, the founder of psychodrama, comes from the one and only time he met Sigmund Freud in person. Moreno shouted across the room at Freud, "You analyze people's dreams. I give them the courage to dream again." Through this book, you have witnessed clients learning to dream again. I hope you have found some dreams and visions of your future as well. Go gently.

References

Altman, K. A. (1992). Psychodramatic treatment of multiple personality disorder and dissociative disorders. *Dissociation, 5*(2), 104–108.

Altman, K. P. (1993). Psychodrama in the treatment of post-abuse syndromes. *Treating Abuse Today, 2,* 27–31.

Altman, K. P. (2000). Psychodramatic treatment of multiple personality disorder and dissociative disorders. In P. F. Kellermann & M. K. Hudgins (Eds.), *Psychodrama with trauma survivors: Acting out your pain* (pp. 179–186). London: Jessica Kingsley Publishers.

American Board of Examiners in Psychodrama, Sociometry and Group Psychotherapy. (1982). *Examination information* [pamphlet]. Washington, DC: Self-published.

American Psychiatric Association. (2000). *Diagnostic and statistical manual of mental disorders* (4th ed.). Washington, DC: APA Books.

Australian and New Zealand Psychodrama Association, Inc. (1989). *Board of Examiners training and standards manual.* Melbourne, Australia: Self-published.

Baim, C. (2000). Time's distorted mirror: Trauma work with adult male sex offenders. In P. F. Kellermann & M. K. Hudgins (Eds.), *Psychodrama with trauma survivors: Acting out your pain.* London: Jessica Kingsley Publications.

Bannister, A. (1990). *From hearing to healing: Working with the aftermath of child sexual abuse.* Chichester, United Kingdom: John Wiley.

Bannister, A. (1991). Learning to live again: Psychodramatic techniques with sexually abused young people. In P. Holmes & M. Karp (Eds.), *Psychodrama: Inspiration and technique* (pp. 77–94). London: Tavistock/Routledge.

Bannister, A. (1997). *The healing drama: Psychodrama and drama therapy with abused children.* London: Free Association Books.

Bannister, A. (2000). Prisoners of the family: Psychodrama with abused children. In P. F. Kellermann & M. K. Hudgins (Eds.), *Psychodrama with trauma survivors: Acting out your pain* (pp. 97–113). London: Jessica Kingsley Publishers.

Bannister, A., & Huntington, A. (Eds.). (2002). *Communicating with children and adolescents: Action for change.* London: Jessica Kingsley Publications.

Baratka, C. (1994). *Incorporating the principles of the action trauma team to inpatients with eating disorders* [Monograph]. Charlottesville, VA: Therapeutic Spiral International.

Bass, E., & Davis, L. (1988). *The courage to heal: A guide for women survivors of child sexual abuse.* New York: Harper & Row.

Baumgartner, D. (1986). Sociodrama and the Vietnam combat veteran: A therapeutic release for a wartime experience. *Journal of Group Psychotherapy and Sociometry, 38,* 31–39.

Bergin, A. E., & Garfield, S. L. (Eds.). (1994). *The handbook of psychotherapy and behavior change* (4th ed.). New York: John Wiley & Sons, Inc.

Blatner, A. (1991). Role Dynamics: A comprehensive theory of psychology. *Journal of Group Psychotherapy, Psychodrama and Sociometry, 44*(1), 33–40.

Blatner, A. (1995). Psychodrama. In R. J. Corsini & D. Wedding (Eds.), *Current psychotherapies* (5th ed., pp. 399–408). Itasca, IL: F. E. Peacock.

Blatner, A. (1996). *Acting-in: Practical applications of psychodramatic methods* (3rd ed.). New York: Springer Publishing.

Blatner, A. (1997). Psychodrama: The state of the art. *The Arts in Psychotherapy, 24*(1), 23–30.

Blatner, A. (2000). *Foundations of psychodrama: History, theory, and practice* (4th ed.). New York: Springer Publishing.

British Psychodrama Association. (1993). BPA Training Guidelines. London: Self-published by BPA.

Buchanan, D. R. (1980). The central concern model: A framework for structuring psychodramatic production. *Journal of Group Psychotherapy, Psychodrama and Sociometry, 33,* 47–62.

Buchanan, D. R. (1984). Psychodrama. In T. B. Karasu (Chair), *The psychiatric therapies.* Washington, DC: American Psychiatric Press, Inc.

Burge, M. (1996). The Vietnam veteran and the family "both victims of post traumatic stress"—a psychodramatic perspective. *Australian and New Zealand Psychodrama Association Journal, 5,* 25–36.

Burger, J. B. (1994). *The effects of psychodrama treatment on levels of assertiveness and locus of control in women who have experienced battering.* Unpublished doctoral dissertation, The College of William and Mary.

Carbonell, D. M., & Parteleno-Barehmi, C. (1999). Psychodrama groups for girls coping with trauma. *International Journal of Group Psychotherapy, 49*(3), 285–306.

Chimera, C. (2002). The yellow brick road: Helping children and adolescents to recover a coherent story following abusive family experiences. In A. Bannister & A. Huntington (Eds.), *Communicating with children and adolescents: Action for change.* London: Jessica Kingsley Publications.

Clayton, G. M. (1994). Role theory and its application in clinical practice. In P. Holmes, M. Karp, & M. Watson (Eds.), *Psychodrama since Moreno: Innovation in theory and practice.* London: Routledge.

Clayton, L. (1982). The use of the cultural atom to record personality change in individual psychotherapy. *Journal of Group Psychotherapy, Psychodrama and Sociometry, 35,* 111–117.

Cornell, W. F., & Olio, K. A. (1991). Integrating affect in treatment with adult survivors of physical and sexual abuse. *American Journal of Orthopsychiatry, 61*(1), 59–69.

Cossa, M. (1999). Doodah management. The Center for Experiential Learning newsletter, p. 1–2. Now available at Therapeutic Spiral International, Charlottesville, Virginia.

Cossa, M. (2000). *The doodah song.* The Center for Experiential Learning (Charlottesville, VA) Newsletter (Winter). Available now from Therapeutic Spiral International.

Cossa, M. (2002). Drago-drama: Archetypal sociodrama with adolescents. In A. Bannister & A. Huntington (Eds.), *Communicating with children and adolescents: Action for change.* London: Jessica Kingsley Publications.

Cossa, M., & Hudgins, M. K. (1998). *Workshop handout.* Keene, NH: ACTINGOUT.

Courtois, C. A. (1988). *Healing the incest wound: Adult survivors in therapy.* New York: W. W. Norton.

Culbertson, R. (2001). *Sacred bearings: A journal on violence and spiritual life.* Charlottesville, VA: University of Virginia.

Dayton, T. (1994). *The drama within: Psychodrama and experiential therapy.* Deerfield Beach, FL: Health Communications, Inc.

Dayton, T. (1997). *Heartwounds: Unresolved grief and trauma.* Deerfield Beach, FL: Health Communications, Inc.

Dayton, T. (2000a). *Trauma and addiction.* Deerfield Beach, FL: Health Communications, Inc.

Dayton, T. (2000b). The use of psychodrama in the treatment of trauma and addiction. In P. F. Kellermann & M. K. Hudgins (Eds.), *Psychodrama with trauma survivors: Acting out your pain.* London: Jessica Kingsley Publications.

Dogner, I., & Valip, I. (1994). Sociometric and psychodramatic group therapy with bipolar patients [Turkish]. *Tuerk Psikiyatri Dergisi, 5*(2), 127–133.

Eckert, J., & Biermann-Ratjen, E.-M. (1998). The treatment of borderline personality disorder. In L. S. Greenberg, J. C. Watson, & G. Lietaer (Eds.), *Handbook of experiential psychotherapy* (pp. 349–367). New York: Guilford Press.

Ellenson, G. S. (1986). Disturbances of perception in adult female incest survivors. *Journal of Contemporary Social Work, 67,* 149–159.

Ellenson, G. S. (1989). Horror, rage and defenses in the symptoms of female sexual abuse survivors. *Social Casework: The Journal of Contemporary Social Work,* (December), 589–598.

Elliot, R., Davis, K. L., & Slatick, E. (1998). Process-experiential therapy for posttraumatic stress difficulties. In L. S. Greenberg, J. C. Watson, & G. Lietaer (Eds.), *Handbook of experiential psychotherapy* (pp. 249–271). New York: Guilford Press.

Elliott, R., Greenberg, L. S., & Lietaer, G. (2002). Research on experiential therapies. In M. Lambert, A. Bergin, & S. Garfield (Eds.), *Handbook of psychotherapy and behavior change* (5th ed.). New York: John Wiley & Sons, Inc.

Elliot, R., Suter, P., Manford, J., Radpour-Markert, L., Siegel-Hinson, R., Layman, C., & Davis, K. (1996). A process-experiential approach to post-traumatic stress disorder. In R. Hutter, G. Pawlowsky, P. F. Schmid, & R. Stipsits (Eds.), *Client-centered and experiential psychotherapy: A paradigm in motion* (pp. 235–254). Frankfurt am Main: Lang.

Farmer, C. (1998). The psychodramatic treatment of depression. In M. Karp, P. Holmes, & K. B. Tauvon (Eds.), *The handbook of psychodrama.* London: Routledge.

Forst, M. (2001). *The Therapeutic Spiral Model: A qualitative enquiry of its effectiveness in the treatment of trauma and addiction.* Unpublished manuscript, University of Ottawa.

Fox, J. (Ed.). (1987). *The essential Moreno: Writings on psychodrama, group method and spontaneity by J. L. Moreno.* New York: Springer Publishing.

Friedman, N. (1976). From experiential in therapy to experiential in psychotherapy: A history. *Psychotherapy: Theory, Research and Practice, 13*(3), 236–243.

Fuhlrodt, R. L. (Ed.). (1990). *Psychodrama: Its application to ACOA and substance abuse treatment.* East Rutherford, NJ: Thomas W. Perin, Inc.

Gelinas, D. J. (1983). The persisting negative effects of incest. *Psychiatry, 46,* 312–332.

Gendlin, E. T. (1962). *Experiencing and the creation of meaning: A philosophical and psychological approach to the subjective.* New York: Free Press of Glencoe.

Gendlin, E. T. (1996). *Focusing-oriented psychotherapy: A manual of the experiential method.* New York: Guilford Press.

Goldman, E. E., & Morrison, D. S. (1984). *Psychodrama: Experience and process.* Dubuque, IA: Kendall/Hunt.

Greenberg, L. S. (2001). *Emotion-focussed therapy: Coaching clients to work through feelings.* Washington, DC: American Psychological Association Press.

Greenberg, L. S., Elliott, R. K., & Lietaer, G. (1994). Research on experiential psychotherapies. In A. E. Bergin & S. L. Garfield (Eds.), *Handbook of psychotherapy and behavior change* (4th ed., pp. 509–539). New York: John Wiley & Sons, Inc.

Greenberg, L. S., Korman, L., & Paivio, S. C. (2001). Emotion in humanistic therapy. In D. Cain & J. Seeman (Eds.), *Humanistic psychotherapies: Handbook of research and practice.* Washington, DC: American Psychological Association Press.

Greenberg, L. S., & Paivio, S. C. (1997). *Working with emotions in psychotherapy.* New York: Guilford Press.

Greenberg, L. S., & Paivio, S. C. (1998). Allowing and accepting painful emotional experiences. *The International Journal of Action Methods, 51*(2), 47–62.

Greenberg, L. S., Rice, L. N., & Elliott, R. K. (1993). *Facilitating emotional change: The moment-by-moment process.* New York: Guilford Press.

Greenberg, L. S., & Van Balen, R. (1998). The theory of experience-centered therapies. In L. S. Greenberg, J. C. Watson, & G. Lietaer (Eds.), *Handbook of experiential psychotherapy* (pp. 28–57). New York: Guilford Press.

Greenberg, L. S., Watson, J. C., & Goldman, R. (1998). Process-experiential therapy in depression. In L. S. Greenberg, J. C. Watson, & G. Lietaer (Eds.), *Handbook of experiential psychotherapy* (pp. 227–248). New York: Guilford Press.

Greenberg, L. S., Watson, J. C., & Lietaer, G. (Eds.). (1998). *Handbook of experiential psychotherapy.* New York: Guilford Press.

Hale, A. (1985). *Conducting clinical sociometric explorations* (Rev. ed.). Roanoke, VA: Royal Publishing Company.

Haworth, P. (1998). The historical background of psychodrama. In M. Karp, P. Holmes, & K. B. Tauvon (Eds.), *The handbook of psychodrama.* London: Routledge.

Herman, J. L. (1992a). *Trauma and recovery.* New York: Basic Books.

Herman, J. L. (1992b). Complex PTSD: A syndrome in survivors of prolonged and repeated trauma. *Journal of Traumatic Stress, 5,* 377–391.

Hollander, C. (1969). *A process for psychodrama training: The Hollander psychodrama curve* [monograph]. Denver, CO: Evergreen Institute Press.

Holmes, P. (1991). Classical psychodrama: An overview. In P. Holmes & M. Karp (Eds.), *Psychodrama: Inspiration and technique* (pp. 7–14). London: Tavistock/Routledge.

Holmes, P. (1992). *The inner world outside: Object relations theory and psychodrama.* London: Tavistock/Routledge.

Holmes, P., & Karp, M. (Eds.). (1991). *Psychodrama: Inspiration and technique.* London: Tavistock/Routledge.

Holmes, P., Karp, M., & Watson, M. (Eds.). (1994). *Psychodrama since Moreno: Innovations in theory and practice.* London: Routledge.

Hudgins, M. K. (1989). Experiencing the self through psychodrama and gestalt therapy in anorexia nervosa. In L. M. Hornyak & E. R. Baker (Eds.), *Experiential therapies for eating disorders* (pp. 234–251). New York: Guilford Press.

Hudgins, M. K. (1993). Videotape: Healing sexual trauma with action methods. Madison, WI: Digital Recordings. (Available from Therapeutic Spiral International.)

Hudgins, M. K. (1998). Experiential psychodrama with sexual trauma. In L. S. Greenberg, J. C. Watson, & G. Lietaer (Eds.), *Handbook of experiential psychotherapy* (pp. 328–348). New York: Guilford Press.

Hudgins, M. K. (2000). The therapeutic spiral model: Treating PTSD in action. In P. F. Kellermann & M. K. Hudgins (Eds.), *Psychodrama with trauma survivors: Acting out your pain.* London: Jessica Kingsley Publications.

Hudgins, M. K., & Drucker, K. (1998). The containing double as part of the Therapeutic Spiral Model for treating trauma survivors. *The International Journal of Action Methods, 51*(2), 63–74.

Hudgins, M. K., Drucker, K., & Metcalf, K. (1998). *Instructional manual for the intervention module of the containing double* [Monograph]. Charlottesville, VA: Therapeutic Spiral International.

Hudgins, M. K., Drucker, K., & Metcalf, K. (2000). The containing double: A clinically effective psychodrama intervention for PTSD. *The British Journal of Psychodrama and Sociodrama, 15*(1), 58–77.

Hudgins, M. K., & Kellermann, P. F. (2000). Introduction. In P. F. Kellermann & M. K. Hudgins (Eds.), *Psychodrama with trauma survivors: Acting out your pain* (pp. 11–22). London: Jessica Kingsley Publishers.

Hudgins, M. K., & Kiesler, D. J. (1987). Individual experiential psychotherapy: An analogue validation of the intervention module of psychodramatic doubling. *Psychotherapy, 24*(2), 245–255.

Hudgins, M. K., & Kipper, D. A. (1998). Introduction: Action methods in the treatment of trauma survivors. *The International Journal of Action Methods, 51*(2), 43–46.

Hug, E. (1997). Current trends in psychodrama: Eclectic and analytic dimensions. In *Arts in Psychotherapy, 24*, 31–35.

Karp, M. (1991). Psychodrama and piccalilli: Residential treatment of a sexually abused adult. In P. Holmes & M. Karp (Eds.), *Psychodrama: Inspiration and technique* (pp. 95–114). London: Tavistock/Routledge.

Karp, M., Holmes, P., & Tauvon, K. B. (Eds.). (1998). *The handbook of psychodrama.* London: Routledge.

Kellermann, P. F. (1992). *Focus on psychodrama: The therapeutic aspects of psychodrama.* London: Jessica Kingsley Publishers.

Kellermann, P. F. (1996). Concretization in psychodrama with somatization disorder. *The Arts in Psychotherapy, 23,* 149–152.

Kellermann, P. F. (2000). The therapeutic aspects of psychodrama with traumatized people. In P. F. Kellermann & M. K. Hudgins (Eds.), *Psychodrama with trauma survivors: Acting out your pain* (pp. 23–40). London: Jessica Kingsley Publishers.

Kellerman, P. F., & Hudgins, M. K. (Eds.). (2000). *Psychodrama with trauma survivors: Acting out your pain.* London: Jessica Kingsley Publishers.

Kipper, D. A. (1997). Classical and contemporary psychodrama: A multifaceted, action-oriented psychotherapy. *The International Journal of Action Methods, 50*(3), 99–107.

Kipper, D. A. (2000). Spontaneity: Does the experience match the theory? *The International Journal of Action Methods, 53*(1), 33–47.

Leutz, G. A. (2000). Appearance and treatment of dissociative states of consciousness in psychodrama. In P. F. Kellermann & M. K. Hudgins (Eds.), *Psychodrama with trauma survivors: Acting out your pain* (pp. 187–197). London: Jessica Kingsley Publishers.

Leveton, E. (1977/1992). *A clincian's guide to psychodrama.* New York: Springer.

McVea, C. S. (1997). *Moving from isolation to relatedness: The application of psychodramatic theory and techniques when working with a "lone warrior" in one-to-one therapy.* Unpublished thesis (monograph). Brisbane, Australia: Queensland Training Institute.

Mehdi, P. R., Sen, M. D. P., & Sen, A. K. (1997). The usefulness of psychodrama in the treatment of depressed patients. *Indian Journal of Clinical Psychology, 24*(1), 82–92.

Miller, C. (2000). The technique of Souldrama and its applications. *The International Journal of Action Methods, 52*(4), 173–186.

Moreno, J. L. (1920). *Das testament des vaters* [Words of the father]. Berlin: Gustav Kiepenheuer Verlag. (In English, New York: Beacon House, 1941; 1971.)

Moreno, J. L. (1947/1973). *Theatre of spontaneity* (2nd ed.). Beacon, NY: Beacon House, Inc.

Moreno, J. L. (1953). *Who shall survive?* Beacon, NY: Beacon House, Inc.

Moreno, J. L. (1961). The role concept, a bridge between psychiatry and sociology. *American Journal of Psychiatry, 188,* 518–523.

Moreno, J. L. (1965). Therapeutic vehicles and the concept of surplus reality. *Group Psychotherapy, 18*(4), 211–216.

Moreno, J. L. (1977). *Psychodrama* (Vol. 1). Beacon, NY: Beacon House, Inc. (Original work published 1946)

Moreno, J. L., & Moreno, Z. T. (1969). *Psychodrama* (Vol. 3). Beacon, NY: Beacon House, Inc.

Moreno, Z. T. (1959). A survey of psychodramatic techniques. *Group Psychotherapy, 12,* 5–14.

Moreno, Z. T. (1965). Psychodramatic rules, techniques and adjunctive methods. *Group Psychotherapy, 18*(1–2), 73–86.

Moreno, Z. T., Blomkvist, L. D., & Rützel, T. (2000). *Psychodrama, surplus reality and the art of healing.* London: Routledge.

Raaz, N., Carlson-Sabelli, L., & Sabelli, H. (1993). Psychodrama in the treatment of multiple personality disorder: A process-theory perspective. In E. Kluft (Ed.), *Expressive and functional therapies in the treatment of multiple personality disorder.* Springfield, IL: Charles Thomas.

Ragsdale, K. G., Cox, R. D., Finn, P., & Eisler, R. M. (1996). Effectiveness of short-term specialized inpatient treatment for war-related posttraumatic stress disorder: A role for adventure-based counselling and psychodrama. *Journal of Traumatic Stress, 9*(2), 269–283.

Rawlinson, J. (2000). Does psychodrama work? A review of the literature. *The British Journal of Psychodrama and Sociodrama, 15*(2), 67–102.

Remer, R. (2000). Secondary victims of trauma: Producing secondary survivors. In P. F. Kellermann & M. K. Hudgins (Eds.), *Psychodrama with trauma survivors: Acting out your pain* (pp. 317–339). London: Jessica Kingsley Publishers.

Reynolds, T. (1996). Dissociative identity disorder and the psychodramatist. *Australian and New Zealand Psychodrama Association Journal, 5,* 43–61.

Rezaeian, M. P., Mazumdar, D. P. S., & Sen, A. K. (1997). The effectiveness of psychodrama in changing the attitudes among depressed patients. *Journal of Personality and Clinical Studies, 13*(1–2), 19–23.

Ridge, R. M. (1998). Rebuilding the body of trust. The Center for Experiential Learning (Charlottesville, VA) Newsletter (Winter). Available at Therapeutic Spiral International.

Robson, M. (2000). Psychodrama with adolescent sexual offenders. In P. F. Kellermann & M. K. Hudgins (Eds.), *Psychodrama with trauma survivors: Acting out your pain.* London: Jessica Kingsley Publications.

Rustin, T. A., & Olson, P. A. (1993). A variation on Magic Shop for addiction treatment patients. *Journal of Group Psychotherapy, Psychodrama and Sociometry, 46*(1), 12–23.

Schore, A. N. (1994). *Affect regulation and the origin of the self: The neurobiology of emotional development.* Hillsdale, NJ: Lawrence Erlbaum.

Schore, A. N. (1997). The neurodevelopmental aspects of projective identification. Paper presented at the National Conference on Psychoanalysis in Clinical Social Work, Seattle, Washington.

Sheridan, M. S., & Hudgins, M. K. (1990). *The Three-Child Model of Recovery.* Unpublished manuscript, Virginia Commonwealth University, Richmond, VA. Available at Therapeutic Spiral International.

Sidorsky, S. (1984). The psychodramatic treatment of the borderline personality. *Journal of Group Psychotherapy, Psychodrama and Sociometry, 37,* 117–125.

Slavson, S. R. (1951). Catharsis in group psychotherapy. *Psychoanalytic Review, 38,* 39–52.

Terr, L. C. (1991). Childhood traumas: An outline and overview. *American Journal of Psychiatry, 148*(1), 10–20.

Tomasulo, D. J. (2001). Culture in action: Diversity training with a cultural double. *The International Journal of Action Methods, 53*(2), 51–65.

Toscani, M. F. (1993). *The wholeness of the action trauma team: The shared director's role* [monograph]. Charlottesville, VA: The Center for Experiential Learning. (Available now from Therapeutic Spiral International.)

Toscani, M. F., & Hudgins, M. K. (1996). *Trauma survivor's intrapsychic role atom: Including prescriptive roles* [Monograph]. Charlottesville, VA: The Center for Experiential Learning. (Available now from Therapeutic Spiral International.)

Turner, S. W., McFarlane, A. C., & van der Kolk, B. A. (1996). The therapeutic environment and new explorations in the treatment of posttraumatic stress disorder. In B. A. van der Kolk, A. C. McFarlane, & L. Weisaeth (Eds.), *Traumatic stress: The effects of overwhelming experience on mind, body, and society* (pp. 537–558). New York: Guilford Press.

van der Kolk, B. A. (1996a). The complexity of adaptation to trauma: Self-regulation, stimulus discrimination, and characterological development. In B. A. van der Kolk, A. C. McFarlane, & L. Weisaeth (Eds.), *Traumatic stress: The effects of overwhelming experience on mind, body, and society* (pp. 182–213). New York: Guilford Press.

van der Kolk, B. A. (1996b). The body keeps score: Approaches to the psychobiology of posttraumatic stress disorder. In B. A. van der Kolk, A. C. McFarlane, & L. Weisaeth (Eds.), *Traumatic stress: The effects of overwhelming experience on mind, body, and society* (pp. 214–241). New York: Guilford Press.

van der Kolk, B. A. (1997a). The psychobiology of post-traumatic stress disorder. *Journal of Clinical Psychiatry, 58*(Suppl. 9).

van der Kolk, B. (1997b, February). *Keynote address.* Presented at the annual conference of the American Society of Group Psychotherapy and Psychodrama, New York, NY.

Van der Kolk, B. A., & McFarlane, A. C. (1996). The black hole of trauma. In B. A. van der Kolk, A. C. McFarlane, & L. Weisaeth (Eds.), *Traumatic stress: The effects of overwhelming experience on mind, body, and society* (pp. 3–23). New York: The Guilford Press.

van der Kolk, B. A., McFarlane, A. C., & Weisaeth, L. (Eds.). (1996). *Traumatic stress: The effects of overwhelming experience on mind, body, and society.* New York: Guilford Press.

van der Kolk, B. A., van der Hart, O., & Marmar, C. R. (1996). Dissociation and information processing in posttraumatic stress disorder. In B. A. van der Kolk, A. C. McFarlane, & L. Weisaeth (Eds.), *Traumatic stress: The effects of overwhelming experience on mind, body, and society* (pp. 303–327). New York: Guilford Press.

Watson, J. C., Greenberg, L. S., & Lietaer, G. (1998). The experiential paradigm unfolding: Relationship and experiencing in therapy. In L. S. Greenberg, J. C. Watson, & G. Lietaer (Eds.), *Handbook of experiential psychotherapy* (pp. 3–27). New York: Guilford Press.

Widlake, B. (1997). Barbara's bubbles: The psychodrama of a young adult recovering from an eating disorder. *The British Journal of Psychodrama and Sociodrama, 12,* 23–34.

Wilkins, P. (1997). Psychodrama and research. *The British Journal of Psychodrama and Sociodrama, 12,* 44–61.

Winters, N. L. (2000). The psychospiritual in psychodrama: A fourth role category. *The International Journal of Action Methods, 52*(1), 163–172.

Wolf, B. E., & Sigl, P. (1998). Experiential psychotherapy of the anxiety disorders. In L. S. Greenberg, J. C. Watson, & G. Lietaer (Eds.), *Handbook of experiential psychotherapy* (pp. 272–294). New York: Guilford Press.

Young, L. (1992). Sexual abuse and the problem of embodiment. *Child Abuse and Neglect, 16,* 89–100.

Diagnostic Criteria for Posttraumatic Stress Disorder

A. The person has been exposed to a traumatic event in which both of the following were present:

   1) The person experienced, witnessed, or was confronted with an event or events that involved actual or threatened death or serious injury, or a threat to the physical integrity of self or others.

   2) The person's response involved intense fear, helplessness, or horror. *Note:* In children, this may be expressed instead by disorganized or agitated behavior.

B. The traumatic event is persistently reexperienced in one (or more) of the following ways:

   1) Recurrent and intrusive distressing recollections of the event, including images, thoughts, or perceptions. *Note:* In young children, repetitive play may occur in which themes or aspects of the trauma are expressed.

   2) Recurrent distressing dreams of the event. *Note:* In children, there may be frightening dreams without recognizable content.

   3) Acting or feeling as if the traumatic event were recurring (includes a sense of reliving the experience, illusions, hallucinations, and dissociative flashback episodes, including those that occur upon awakening or when intoxicated). *Note:* In young children, trauma-specific reenactment may occur.

   4) Intense psychological distress at exposure to internal or external cues that symbolize or resemble an aspect of the traumatic event.

   5) Physiological reactivity at exposure to internal or external cues that symbolize or resemble an aspect of the traumatic event.

C. Persistent avoidance of stimuli associated with the trauma and numbing of general responsiveness (not present before the trauma) occurs, as indicated by three (or more) of the following:
1) Efforts to avoid thoughts, feelings, or conversations associated with the trauma.
2) Efforts to avoid activities, places, or people that arouse recollections of the trauma.
3) Inability to recall an important aspect of the trauma.
4) Markedly diminished interest or participation in significant activities.
5) Feeling of detachment or estrangement from others.
6) Restricted range of affect (e.g., unable to have loving feelings).
7) Sense of a foreshortened future (e.g., does not expect to have a career, marriage, children, or a normal life span).

D. Persistent symptoms of increased arousal (not present before the trauma), as indicated by two (or more) of the following:
1) difficulty falling or staying asleep,
2) irritability or outbursts of anger,
3) difficulty concentrating,
4) hypervigilance, or
5) exaggerated startle response.

E. Duration of the disturbance (symptoms in criteria B, C, and D) is longer than 1 month.

F. The disturbance causes clinically significant distress or impairment in social, occupational, or other important areas of functioning.

Specify whether:
Acute: if duration of symptoms is less than 3 months.
Chronic: if duration of symptoms is 3 months or more.

Specify whether:
With Delayed Onset: if onset of symptoms is at least 6 months after the stressor.

Source: American Psychiatric Association. (2000). *Diagnostic and statistical manual of mental disorders* (4th ed., rev. ed., pp. 467–468). Washington, DC: APA Books.

Glossary of Terms in the Therapeutic Spiral Model

Abandoning authority role: The trauma-based role in the TSIRA that carries the internalization of the traumatic experience where there was no one to help. It is repeated toward self through addictions, eating disorders, lack of self-care, et cetera. It is also acted out toward others as a neglectful parent, or a distant or unfaithful spouse.

Action trauma team: Therapeutic Spiral International builds teams in local communities to use the Therapeutic Spiral Model to treat trauma. They are called action trauma teams because they treat trauma using modified psychodrama methods.

Assistant Leader (AL): The team role that is unique to the Therapeutic Spiral Model. It was created to help manage the integration of group members into a TSM drama when they are triggered. The AL directs all sub-scenes that are outside of the circle of safe experiencing.

Body double (BD): The body double intervention module. This is a prescriptive role from the TSIRA that is used to decrease dissociation and help people experience their bodies in a healthy state.

Change agent: A key transformative role in the TSIRA that serves the function of protecting the self in the here and now from repeating old trauma patterns. It must be enacted prior to anyone reexperiencing their victim, perpetrator, or abandoning authority roles.

Circle of scarves: The TSM action structure that starts off all workshops, groups, and individual sessions. A circle is created out of brightly colored scarves to mark a visual container for trauma material to be enacted within. It is also called the circle of safety or the circle of safe experiencing.

Containing double (CD): The containing double intervention module. This is a prescriptive role from the TSIRA that is used to increase cognitive processing and narrative labeling in the face of trauma material.

Doodah management: This is the term that describes the TSM process to label personal and interpersonal difficulties among action trauma team members. Doodahs are the reactivation of one's own trauma material; defenses such as dissociation or identification with the aggressor, transference, countertransference, acting out—all are signs that a team member's own PTSD is being triggered and must be managed.

Energy: The first strand of the Therapeutic Spiral Model. It is the fuel for all growth and development in TSM. It is defined as a spontaneous state of learning and is activated by enactment of the prescriptive roles of the TSIRA. It also contains a focus on spirituality.

Experiencing: The second strand of TSM. It describes the experiential processes of internal awareness of sensations, perceptions, thoughts, feelings, and actions.

Holder of defenses: A trauma-based role that is enacted to show how rigidly primitive defenses are held in the trauma survivor's intrapsychic role atom.

Intervention module: This describes the clinical enactment of one of the roles that are part of the trauma survivor's intrapsychic role atom. Some interventions are as simple as role reversals. Others have a set of specified and manualized steps for research and training.

Keeper of defenses: A prescriptive role that develops from the interaction of the holder of defenses with the prescriptive roles in a TSM drama. It does what it says—keeps the primitive defenses, such as dissociation, denial, and projective identification. This role makes choices about defenses and seeks to learn new skills for self-organization and interpersonal relationships.

Manager of healthy functioning: A transformative role that develops from the interaction of the keeper of defenses, the change agent role, and the other prescriptive roles. This role goes beyond defenses and finds healthy, adaptive coping skills such as honest communication, trusting intimacy, et cetera.

Meaning: The third strand in the spiral image. It represents the ability to put narrative labels on experience to make sense out of it.

Observing ego (OE): The observing ego intervention module. This is a prescriptive role from the TSIRA that is used to establish a role where people can neutrally observe and narratively label their behaviors.

Perpetrator role: The trauma-based role in the TSIRA that carries the internalization of the violence that was experienced. It is either acted out toward self as self-criticism, shame, self-loathing, or suicide; or it is acted out toward others in the form of murder, abuse, criticism, and blaming.

Prescriptive roles: A set of 8 roles that are prescribed for healthy self-organization for trauma survivors. They always make up Scene 1 in a TSM psychodrama. They include the observing ego; the client role; personal, interpersonal, and transpersonal strengths; the body double; the containing double, and the keeper of defenses.

Principles of Conscious Reexperiencing With Developmental Repair: This is another clinical action structure that is unique to the TSM. It provides six steps in controlled regression:

1) talk,
2) observe,
3) witness,
4) reenact,
5) reexperience, and
6) repair.

Reexperiencing dramas: This is a clinical action structure that is unique to the TSM. Each type of drama provides a contract for clinical goals and boundaries to a drama. There are six types of TSM dramas:

1) Restoration and Renewal,
2) Dreams and Metaphors,
3) Initial Discovery and Accurate Labeling,

4) Uncovering and Exploring Core Trauma,
5) Conscious Reexperiencing With Developmental Repair, and
6) Letting Go and Transformation.

Sleeping-awakening child role: This transformative role was originally developed in the Three Child Model of Recovery (Sheridan & Hudgins, 1990). Now, it is a role in the TSIRA that represents an untouched, innocent, fully alive and vital part of self that was never damaged by traumatic experience.

Team Leader (TL): The clinician who has overall responsibility for directing a TSM drama or workshop.

Therapeutic spiral image: A graphic image of the three strands of the Therapeutic Spiral Model: energy, experiencing, and meaning. It shows all three strands working together in a therapeutic manner.

Therapeutic Spiral International (TSI): This is the nonprofit training institute that provides accreditation in the Therapeutic Spiral Model to treat trauma. It raises funds to bring teams to underserved communities in the global community.

Therapeutic Spiral Model (TSM): The Therapeutic Spiral Model as a whole system of modified psychodrama. This is a trademarked model of experiential change for trauma survivors.

Trained auxiliary ego (TAE): The team role that provides support for a TSM drama. TAEs are trained to enact projective identifications, and the trauma-based roles of victim, perpetrator, and abandoning authority so that group members do not have to do this.

Transformative roles: A set of six roles in the TSIRA, created when the prescriptive roles are added to the trauma-based roles in action. They have the power to change old trauma patterns when enacted in the here and now.

Trauma-based roles: A set of three categories of roles in the TSIRA that result from the internalization of any traumatic experience. Scene 2 of a TSM psychodrama often concretizes defensive structures and introduces the role of keeper of defenses. Further scenes identify, explore, and repair victim, perpetrator, and abandoning authority roles.

Trauma bubbles: A graphic image that was developed as a shorthand symbol to use with clients to describe the experience of cut-off dissociated trauma material that is held in unconscious awareness.

Trauma spiral: A graphic image of the three strands of TSM impacted by trauma. It shows explosions of energy, constriction of experience, and blocked meaning making.

Trauma Survivor's Intrapsychic Role Atom (TSIRA): This is a clinical assessment tool that is unique to the Therapeutic Spiral Model. It is the clinical map that identifies the roles that trauma survivors live with, the healthy, prescriptive roles and the roles required to transform the trauma-based roles, and is the basis for all action interventions in TSM.

Victim role: The trauma-based role in the TSIRA that suffers from the traumatic experience. The word victim is used because it represents the frozen and unprocessed information from the time of trauma.

Wounded child role: The trauma-based role in the TSIRA that reframes the victim role so that unprocessed thoughts, feelings, and actions can be observed, experienced, and expressed.

Overview of the Accreditation Process in the Therapeutic Spiral Model

REQUIREMENTS FOR ENTRY INTO THE TSM ACCREDITATION PROCESS

1. Master's degree and working toward certification in psychodrama or other experiential or expressive arts therapies. *Note:* Candidates who do not possess these qualifications, but have comparable international qualifications, equivalent clinical experience or experiential training, can apply to the Advisory Committee for Training (ACT) for an entry requirements waiver.

2. Participation in at least one TSI Training workshop and one TSI Personal Growth workshop, in which appropriate auxiliary roles are taken as a group member.

3. Recommendation of the Team Leader from the TSI workshop(s) in which the candidate has participated in order to begin the formal TSI training process.

4. Submission to TSI of candidate's curriculum vitae, together with completed and signed Application to Enter the TSM Accreditation Process Form and Request for a Primary Trainer. The Primary Trainer, who must be a TSI Accredited Trainer, will guide the Accreditation candidate through the training process, advising on appropriate workshop and training series choices, supervisory requirements and other training needs.

Before being admitted to the accreditation process, participants are described as being in the Introductory Level within the TSI Accreditation Program.

TRAINING OPTIONS

Having been accepted into the TSI Accreditation Program, there are 3 key routes to achieving TSI Accreditation. The Primary Trainer will usually advise a trainee on which is most suitable. The three routes are as follows:

Participation in a Pre-Scheduled Training Series

Each year, TSI schedules regular Training Series programs on the East and West coasts of the United States, in the United Kingdom, and in Canada, comprised of at least three training workshops. Enrollment in one of these pre-scheduled Training Series requires an up-front commitment of time and money for the entire year. As teams of qualified Associates are built up, the pre-scheduled Training Series program can be extended to new regions and countries.

Participation in Individual Courses on an Ad Hoc Basis

For those whose lifestyle or budget does not fit well with a commitment to an entire year's Training Series, trainees can participate in any of TSI's Training or Personal Growth workshops anywhere in the world on an ad hoc basis. Training on this basis may take more or less than a year, but trainees must have completed a minimum of three training workshops and three practica before being assessed for accreditation at each appropriate level.

Participation in a Group Contract Series

The third training option is for individuals to participate in a Group Contract Series, which may be arranged through their place of work or education. This is a training series arranged by TSI under contract to a specific institution or organization. Under this scenario, the organizing institution may choose to co-fund participant fees either in their entirety or up to a certain amount, or participants may still be required to fund their attendance in full.

LEVELS OF TSI ACCREDITATION

TSI Accreditation can be achieved at four successive levels. Any TSI Action Trauma Team must include Associates fulfilling each of the first three roles, but need not necessarily include a Trainer. The four accreditation levels are described below.

1) Trained Auxiliary Ego (TAE)—The TAE is required to take on any role requested of him/her by the protagonist, Assistant Leader, and/or Team Leader. They may be required to model group trust-building techniques and assist with administrative and team-supportive duties.

2) Assistant Leader (AL)—The AL communicates with all team members prior to workshops and may manage team supervisions during a workshop. S/he is required to maintain an overview of what is going on for all participants and team members in the workshop, and to act as a liaison between them and the team leader. The AL will direct one drama per workshop.

3) Team Leader (TL)—The TL has responsibility for the overall running of a workshop, including budgeting, and for directing the majority of the workshop's dramas. S/he also acts as clinical supervisor for TSI team members. The TL's main focus during the drama is on the protagonist and those working with him/her.

4) Trainer (T)—Trainers are fully versed in all aspects of team roles, trauma theories, and the clinical frameworks that are part of the Therapeutic Spiral Model. They are able to train others in the Model and to build local action trauma teams.

It is not necessary for all trainees to proceed through to Trainer level. Some Associates enjoy working as TAEs on TSI Teams and do not wish to progress to the next level. However, it is necessary for all Associates to maintain a specified level of training and/or involvement each year. Otherwise, they must apply for reaccreditation.

Once Associates are accredited by TSI at any level, they are eligible to participate on TSI Teams in that role for payment. When they are participating on a team in a practicum role, however, they are not eligible for payment.

GENERAL REQUIREMENTS FOR ACCREDITATION AT EACH LEVEL

1. *A minimum of participation in three training workshops and one Personal Growth workshop.* Training workshops are designed to teach participants skills and knowledge relevant to the Therapeutic Spiral

Model. No clients are present. Personal Growth workshops are geared toward healing personal issues, self-development, and renewal.

2.   *Commitment to the practicum process.* This stipulates participation in a minimum of four workshops in the team role for which the applicant is in training. In a trainee's first practicum, s/he will adopt the role s/he is in training for as a back-up. In the following three practica, s/he will participate in the role fully.

3.   *Supervision with a professional approved by a TSI Trainer.* The supervisor need not be affiliated to TSI. A minimum of 20 hours of individual and/or group supervision is required at each level.

4.   *Assessment by one or more Team Leaders or Trainers to the effect that the trainee has demonstrated more than minimum competency during practicum experiences.* Skills checklists of each level are used to support this assessment.

Accreditation candidates should note that each requirement is for a minimum level of achievement. Not all trainees will be ready for accreditation after completing the minimum requirements. It should also be noted that trainees can apply to the Advisory Committee on Training for a waiver of any accreditation requirement, using an Accreditation Waiver Form.

SPECIFIC REQUIREMENTS AT EACH ACCREDITATION LEVEL

LEVEL ONE—TRAINED AUXILIARY EGO (TAE)

1)   A minimum of 100 hours of training and practicum experience in the Therapeutic Spiral Model.
2)   Participation in an Advanced Core Training Series (recommended).
3)   Participation in at least three training workshops and one Personal Growth workshop to complete Level I courses.
4)   Practical demonstration of appropriate role skills on a minimum of four action trauma teams, working directly with clients. On the first practicum, the trainee will act as Backup Auxiliary. S/he must then be a member of at least a further three teams in full Auxiliary Ego role.

5) Demonstration of skills as documented on TAE checklist.
6) A minimum of 20 hours of individual and/or group supervision.

LEVEL TWO—ASSISTANT LEADER (AL)

1) Accreditation as a Trained Auxiliary Ego (TAE).
2) A minimum total of 200 hours of training in the Therapeutic Spiral Model.
3) Participation in an Advanced Core Training Series for at least 1 year.
4) Participation in at least three Training workshops and one Personal Growth workshop to complete Level II courses.
5) Practical demonstration of appropriate role skills on a minimum of four action trauma teams. On the first practicum, the trainee will act as Backup Assistant Leader. S/he must then be a member of at least a further three teams, where an accredited Team Leader or Trainer are present, in full AL role.
6) At least two practica must be on client workshops and one on a training workshop.
7) Organization of at least one local TSI workshop for clients or professionals in which candidate will fulfill AL role.
8) Successful evaluation made by at least two TLs, at least one of whom is a TSM Trainer.
9) Demonstration of skills as documented on the AL checklist.
10) A minimum of 40 hours total of individual and/or group supervision.

LEVEL THREE—TEAM LEADER (TL)

1) Accreditation as an Assistant Leader (AL) and Trained Auxiliary Ego (TAE).
2) A minimum total of 300 hours of training using the Therapeutic Spiral Model.
3) Participation in a Director's Practice or Peer Supervision Group and a TSM personal retreat.
4) If available, participation in a Training Series.
5) Participation in at least three training workshops and one Personal Growth workshop to complete Level III courses.

6) Practical demonstration of appropriate role skills on a minimum five Action Trauma Teams, three of which are pure practica, two of which are assessment practica.

7) On the first practicum, the trainee will share the TL role with an accredited TL. S/he must then be a member of at least a further two teams, where an accredited Team Leader or Trainer is on the team in another role.

8) During the two assessment practica, the trainee takes on the full TL role with a Trainer present and is evaluated for accreditation.

9) Organization of at least one international TSI workshop in which candidate will fulfill TL role.

10) Successful evaluation must be made by at least two TSM Accredited Trainers.

11) Demonstration of skills as documented on the TL checklist.

12) A minimum of 60 total hours of supervision.

LEVEL FOUR—TRAINER (T)

1) Accreditation as a Team Leader (TL) and all other team roles.

2) Completion of Psychodrama, Trainer, Educator, Practitioner (TEP) certification; acceptance into the Practitioner with Application for Trainer (PAT) process or the equivalent by waiver.

3) A minimum total of 400 hours of training using the Therapeutic Spiral Model.

4) Participation in a Trainers' Supervision Group, Training for Trainers Series, and a TSM personal retreat.

5) Practical demonstration of appropriate role skills on a minimum of four training workshops, two of which are pure practica, two of which are assessment practica.

6) On the first practicum, the trainee will share the Trainer role with an accredited Trainer. On the second, the trainee will take on a full Trainer role with an accredited Trainer present.

7) During the two assessment practica, the trainee takes on the full Trainer role with a Trainer present and is evaluated for accreditation.

8) Successful evaluation must be made by at least two TSM Accredited Trainers.

9) Demonstration of skills as documented on the Trainer checklist.

10) A minimum of 80 total hours of individual or group supervision.

REACCREDITATION

Anyone who has been out of TSI work for 18 months or longer needs to be recertified at the highest level for which they were previously accredited. The procedure for this is as follows:

1.   Reaccreditation candidates must participate on one action trauma team in the role of the highest accreditation level they had previously reached. In preparation for this they may participate in a designated reaccreditation weekend training or personal growth workshop.

2.   Once recertified at this highest level, all previously certified lower levels are automatically recertified.

3.   In the event that lower levels were somehow passed over, team members are required to do a practicum to gain those skills.

4.   Accreditation in all team roles (TAE, AL, and TL) is a prerequisite for those seeking to gain Trainer accreditation.

For additional information, please contact

Therapeutic Spiral International
P.O. Box 264
Charlottesville, VA 22902
U.S.A.
Phone: +1-434-923-8290   Toll-free (U.S.): 1-888-475-1615
Fax: +1-434-923-8291
E-mail: mailTSI@aol.com
Direct E-mail: DrKateTSI@aol.com

Index